DEDICATION

To Sheri with love, Julia

To my mother and late father, with love, Craig

ACKNOWLEDGEMENTS

We would like to thank all the health and social care students, teachers and practitioners who have offered insight, advice and help over many years. Our particular thanks go to Sheridan Welsh.

The publishers would like to thank Isabel Dosser, Allison Evans, Joanna McParland, Dr Shaun Speed and David Tait for their insightful review comments on the manuscript and contributions of case studies.

This book is

INTRODUCTION TO PSYCHOLOGY FOR HEALTH CARERS

SECOND EDITION

Julia Russell and Craig Roberts

Australia • Brazil • ⬤ ⬤ gdom • United States

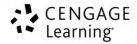

Introduction to Psychology for Health Carers, 2nd Edition
Julia Russell and Craig Roberts

Commissioning Editor Annabel Ainscow

Senior Project Editor: Alison Burt

Manufacturing Buyer: Elaine Willis

Marketing Manager: Sally Gallery

Typesetter: Integra Software Services Pvt. Ltd.

Cover design: Adam Renvoize

For product information and technology assistance,
contact **emea.info@cengage.com.**
For permission to use material from this text or product,
and for permission queries,
email **emea.permissions@cengage.com.**

British Library Cataloguing-in-Publication Data
A catalogue record for this book is available from the British Library.

ISBN: 978-1-4080-8287-4

Cengage Learning EMEA
Cheriton House, North Way, Andover, Hampshire, SP105BE,
United Kingdom

Cengage Learning products are represented in Canada by Nelson Education Ltd.

For your lifelong learning solutions, visit **www.cengage.co.uk**

Purchase your next print book, e-book or e-chapter at
www.cengagebrain.com

Printed in Singapore by Seng Lee Press
1 2 3 4 5 6 7 8 9 10 – 16 15 14

CONTENTS

PREFACE

Health and social care professionals are in constant contact with other people: patients, their visitors and colleagues. The study of psychology, a scientific approach to the understanding of people's thinking and behaviour, can help to enhance the work of health carers. Whether you are just starting out on your career in health care, or you are an established practitioner, this book will help you to understand some of the factors that influence people's decisions and actions. This knowledge will enable you to approach your work in a more professional and effective way.

The content of this book is divided into topics, such as 'communication' and 'stress'. In each chapter the topic is considered from the perspective of both the service user and the health and social care practitioner. This will enable you to gain insight into the issues facing your patients and to envisage ways in which you can improve your own practice.

The book was written after many years of teaching psychology to health and social care students at different levels. Psychology has many uses beyond the classroom and this text intends to show you how the findings of psychological research can help in the practical situations faced by health and social care professionals.

Julia Russell and Craig Roberts

October 2013

ABOUT THE AUTHORS

Julia Russell is a lecturer in the Division of Psychology at Glyndwr University and the Head of Psychology at The Queen's School in Chester.

Craig Roberts is a freelance lecturer and writer in health care and social sciences.

Series Editors for the *Nursing and Health Care Practice* Series:

Dr Lynne Wigens, Director of Nursing and Quality at The Ipswich Hospital NHS Trust; Visiting Senior Fellow University Campus Suffolk.

Dr Jane Day, Head of Division, Practice Learning and Midwifery, School of Nursing and Midwifery, University Campus Suffolk.

INTRODUCTION

The purpose of the book is to provide an introduction to psychology for students on health and social care courses. It aims to present some of the key ideas in psychology that are relevant to health and social care settings. This includes knowledge of general topics within psychology and how these are relevant to improving health and social care and of the process of psychological investigation itself. To this end, the ideas included in each chapter are discussed within the context of up-to-date research. Psychological research can help us to understand the behaviours and problems of patients and staff within the health and social care system and offers insight into ways to help to improve care for patients and staff welfare.

Each chapter has a range of features designed to help you to understand and apply the knowledge presented. The important terms are defined under **keywords** in the margin and are described in more detail in the text. Keywords appear in bold the first time they are used in the text. Each chapter begins with the **learning outcomes**, which will guide you through the text. More complex ideas are described in boxes alongside the text, and some basic psychological ideas are covered in Chapter 1. The central ideas in each chapter are summarized as **key points** throughout the text and an overview is presented in the conclusions at the end of each chapter. You will be encouraged to think about the new ideas and to test your understanding in the **over to you** sections, and **reflective activities** offer you the chance to see how the material you have been working on applies to the health and social care settings that you have experienced. **Case studies** have been taken from real life experiences and illustrate the issues that each chapter is dealing with. Psychology in action in the health and social care environment is illustrated in the **student speaks** and **Professional speaks** features. The **research in brief** boxes provide a summary of evidence-based investigations about the topic. Finally, **rapid recap** questions at the end of each chapter enable you to test your knowledge.

Digital Support Resources

All of our Higher Education textbooks are accompanied by a range of digital support resources. Each title's resources are carefully tailored to the specific needs of the particular book's readers. Examples of the kind of resources provided include:

- Self-test questions
- PowerPoint slides
- Additional references

Lecturers: to discover the dedicated lecturer digital support resources accompanying this textbook please register here for access: **http://login.cengage.com**

Students: to discover the dedicated student digital support resources accompanying this textbook, please search for *Introduction to Psychology for Health Carers* second edition on: **www.cengagebrain.com**

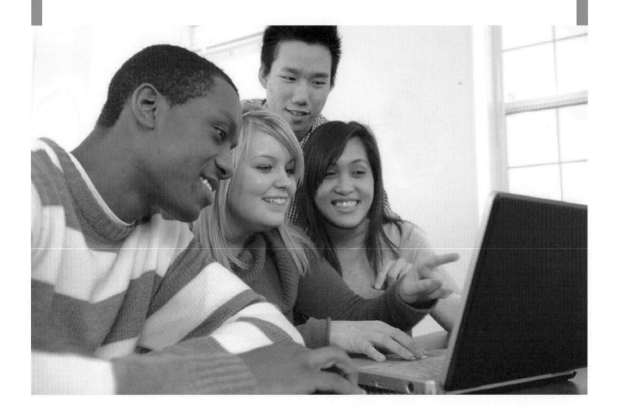

CHAPTER 1
INTRODUCTION

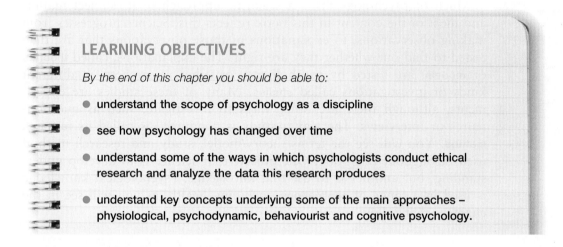

LEARNING OBJECTIVES

By the end of this chapter you should be able to:

- understand the scope of psychology as a discipline

- see how psychology has changed over time

- understand some of the ways in which psychologists conduct ethical research and analyze the data this research produces

- understand key concepts underlying some of the main approaches – physiological, psychodynamic, behaviourist and cognitive psychology.

WHAT IS PSYCHOLOGY?

A simple definition of psychology is 'the scientific study of the mind and behaviour', which includes not just understanding aspects of observable actions, but also making inferences about unobservable constructs, such as memory and emotion. Proposing and testing theories, to make sure they are effective models of human behaviour and thinking, is important as psychologists want to make use of what they discover and apply the findings to real life problems, such as the world of health and social care.

Unlike other subjects, biology for example, it isn't easy to mark out the territory of psychology. This problem arises for several interconnected reasons. Psychology is a bit 'fuzzy at the edges'. Some areas border on other disciplines, such as the biological aspects of stress or the social aspects of prejudice. Because humans are so complex, explanations of our thinking and behaviour are necessarily wide-ranging, hence there has been a spread of ways to explore and interpret what has been observed. This has resulted in many different 'paradigms', or ways of thinking about psychological phenomena.

Over time, different types of explanations have been favoured and this has resulted in a number of approaches or perspectives in psychology. As a result, and in contrast to other sciences, psychology doesn't yet have a single, underlying set of principles. This makes it different from, chemistry, for example, which explains all its phenomena from the standpoint of there being lots of types of 'building blocks', the elements, which are joined together by bonds to make different molecules. Differences in these elements and bonds are the foundation for understanding the whole subject. In psychology there are many ways of looking at what the 'building blocks' might be and how they interact. This is why there are different approaches. We will take a brief historical tour of psychology to look at some of those approaches in the next section.

Much of psychology takes a scientific approach to its subject matter, and most of the content in this book reflects this. Science progresses from making observations, to explanations of those observations that are then tested to find out whether they are right. The explanations, called theories or models, are tested by psychologists or other researchers, in different kinds of investigations called studies. Many of these studies are experiments, although there are other ways to investigate, such as questionnaires or interviews. The way a study is conducted is called its research method. You will see the terms theory/model, study and research method used throughout this book. One objective of science is to develop understanding, but another is to use that knowledge. Psychological knowledge is used in a range of applications, including health, as you will see in the chapters that follow.

A BRIEF HISTORY OF PSYCHOLOGY

Before we start to consider the range of perspectives, it is useful to think about what, exactly, psychology is trying to explain. One helpful idea is 'CAB' (or 'ABC') this aims to remind you of three aspects of the human experience:

- Cognitive
- Affective (emotional)
- Behavioural.

This can be used to understand many different aspects of psychology of the human experience, such as prejudice or grief. We could consider the example of grief in several different ways:

- a grieving person *thinks* about their loved one, tries to *understand* why they have died (a *cognitive* process)
- a grieving person *feels* unhappy (an *affective* response)
- a grieving person may *withdraw* or *cry* (a *behavioural* response).

These ideas can help you to see how psychologists exploring the same phenomenon can do so through different perspectives.

Theory or model
An explanation which helps to understand, predict and potentially control a phenomenon. It can be refined by proposing hypotheses and testing them in studies

Study
An investigation used to explore a phenomenon using one of a range of research methods

Research method
The way a study is conducted, for example using experiments, questionnaires, interviews or a case study

Application
A way to use the findings of a study or the understanding derived from a theory in the world in a practical way

The earliest psychologists

Several people, working independently in different countries began to look at aspects of what we now call psychology. Among them was the physiologist Wilhelm Wundt who, in Germany in 1879, set up the first psychology laboratory. There, he began studying the workings of the mind through observing the nature of one's own experiences, such as thoughts, perceptions and feelings. This is called introspection. He recorded these observations in systematic ways, for example using controlled exposure to a stimulus and measuring the response. Many of the aspects of Wundt's approach (e.g. controls and accurate measurements) laid the scientific foundations of psychology.

Introspection
A way to study psychology through self-analysis

Stimulus
Something, such as an event, object or person, which motivates us to make a response

Control
An imposed standardization, which reduces unwanted variation, allowing the researcher to be sure that changes in the variable they are studying have not been caused by random fluctuations in the internal or external environment of the participant

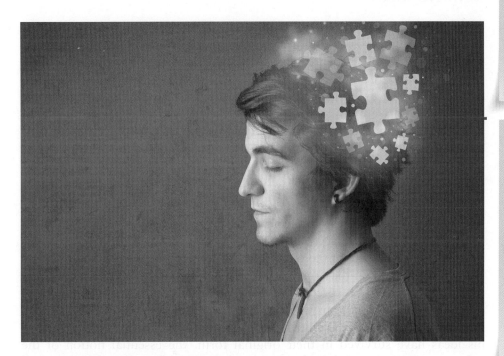

Psychology typically concentrates on internal aspects of *the individual.*

Around the same time, Charles Darwin published 'The Origin of Species', his book on the theory of evolution by natural selection. His focus, explaining that behaviours come about because they are of benefit, influenced William James, a psychologist, who suggested that since human consciousness had evolved, it too must serve a useful function. Unlike Wundt, who was interested in the mental *structures* associated with experiences he observed, James was interested in how the mind *functioned.*

These two contrasting approaches, focusing on structure and function in psychology were initially competing viewpoints but have been progressively replaced by other ways of exploring our conscious experience.

Physiological psychology

Around the start of the 20th Century many psychologists, like Wundt, were investigating biological processes as a way to explore psychological phenomena such as emotional states and stress. Studies of fear identified the role of the spinal cord in transmitting messages from the tissue and organs to the brain, for example about how fast our heart is beating. Both the nervous system and hormones were shown to be involved in our response to stress. Such investigations could be done in a practical way, so were much more scientific than the use of introspection.

Behaviourism

Another group of psychologists using scientific methods to study psychology at the turn of the 20th Century, were the behaviourists. Beginning with Pavlov (in Russia) and Thorndike, Watson and then Skinner in the USA, behaviourists were interested in explaining how new behaviours arose. To ensure that their explorations were scientific, they studied only observable phenomena, so were limited to observing the triggers of behaviour (stimuli) and their consequences (responses), hence the approach is sometimes referred to as S–R psychology.

Freud and psychodynamic psychology

Through the physiological and behaviourist approaches, psychologists could study only material structures and events. Sigmund Freud, in contrast, was interested in the aspect of the mind that could not be seen – the unconscious. He wanted to explain the origins of the personality and how mental illnesses arose so they could be cured. Freud, the founding father of psychoanalysis, developed a vast body of psychological theory, using concepts relating to the unconscious mind and the influences of our early childhood. Although few of his ideas have survived in their original form, the essential notion of the existence of a realm of thought outside our conscious awareness is accepted and still studied.

Cognitive psychology

In some respects, the behaviourists' study of exclusively observable phenomena on one hand, and Freud's explorations of the entirely hidden unconscious on the other, were polar extremes. What was needed was a way to explore hidden aspects of thinking in scientific ways. In the post-war years this became possible as advancements in technology provided both equipment with which to study the mind and a model of how it might work – the computer. The new approach to psychology that emerged, the cognitive approach, looks at the ways in which we process information. It therefore includes attention, perception, thinking, problem solving memory and language and tackles these topics largely through experiments. In comparison to behaviourism, cognitive psychology studies what might be happening between the appearance of the stimulus and the generation of the response. For example, cognitive psychologists look at the factors that might affect a person's recall (their response) of information about how to perform exercises following an operation (the stimulus). These cognitive factors might include repetition or the way they try to remember, such as thinking about the exercises as a dance, or memorizing the order of movements.

Social psychology

Another product of the post-war years was an interest in social psychology, looking for explanations for the atrocities that had been seen. This domain of psychology explored such areas as obedience (following orders), compliance (following the behaviour of the group), the formation of stereotypes and prejudice. Whilst it is more difficult to perform laboratory studies in social psychology, experiments are an important way to study this field.

Psychology today

All of the ideas we have mentioned above still form an active part of the body of research that psychology encompasses. However, the current trend is towards cognitive neuroscience, the idea that we can explain behaviours in terms of how the brain controls mental processes. In part this has been made possible by another advancement in technology – brain scanning – although this is by no means the only weapon in the armoury of the cognitive neuroscientists.

HOW DO PSYCHOLOGISTS CONDUCT STUDIES?

Remember that psychology is the *scientific* study of the mind and behaviour. Psychologists use a range of different ways to explore the phenomena they study, this section explores some of these and how they are used to generate data to test theories.

In order to ensure that these investigations are scientific, rigorous controls are put in place. Psychologists also have to conduct studies in a way that is ethically acceptable, that is with due attention to the welfare of the participants. The ways in which these two, sometimes contradictory objectives are achieved is also considered.

What makes a scientifically good study?

Validity and reliability

There are many concepts that can be used to judge the effectiveness of a study. Two very important ones are reliability and validity.

Reliability

This is a judgment of whether a 'measure', such as a task or test, produces similar results each time it is used in a similar situation. For example, would a patient give the same answer to the question 'Are you feeling better today?' if tested twice? An unreliable measure is not useful as it cannot be trusted.

Reliability may depend on how and who takes measures. Consider an example of measuring pain. If two nurses observed a patient and one recorded behaviours, such as frowning and wincing (indicating pain), but the other recorded the patient getting up to the toilet and feeding herself, they would come to different conclusions about the patient pain, so their findings would not be reliable. Even if both nurses recorded facial expressions, one might focus on frowning and the other on smiling, again they would come to different conclusions, i.e. their results would be unreliable.

Scientific instruments, such as thermometers and sphygmomanometers are more reliable than psychological measures, such as those based on questionnaires or interviews. Here, researchers try to ensure that reliability is high by making sure that there are clear definitions and procedures to follow when testing participants and recording data.

Validity

This is a judgment about whether a measure or manipulation really does assess or deliberately change what it claims to, rather than some other factor. Looking at the measurement of pain again; does a measure really assess pain or something different, such as the tendency of the individual to appeal for sympathy, or fear of pain and consequent requests for analgesia. If two independent measures of a variable, such as a questionnaire and an observation, report similar levels of the variable, they are considered to be valid. Similarly, if researchers intend to compare two alternative treatments, they must be certain that the only difference between treatments they are comparing are the intended ones. For example, in a comparison of the efficacy of nurse-led compared to GP-led advice for asthmatics, it is important that the participants receiving advice in each group are given the same information, spend the same amount of time being supervized and are both offered the chance to ask questions.

Threats to validity and reliability

Subjectivity versus objectivity

In addition to being reliable and valid, an effective study must also fairly reflect the response of the participant, rather than just the view of the researcher. This is the need for objectivity over subjectivity.

Subjectivity is a bias caused by an individual's personal perspective. For example, if the report from a patient's own GP differed from the view of a clinician observing the patient for the first time, the difference may be due to the patient's own GP having a long-standing involvement with that individual's care.

Objectivity, in contrast, refers to an independent perspective, one that does not have the self as a point of reference. Consider how a practice nurse might find out about how well a new treatment regime is working for a patient with a chronic condition. Asking the patient how they are getting on is important, it will inform the nurse about the patient's attitude to the treatment – are they confident, anxious, satisfied, etc. but the answers will be subjective. Perhaps the treatment is more effective than the patient perceives because they are doubtful as nothing has worked before. More objective ways to find out might include taking the blood pressure of a patient on antihypertensives or measuring the blood glucose level of a diabetic. These measures are independent of the personal viewpoints of either the patient or the nurse.

A range of techniques in research help to maximize objectivity, including 'blind' procedures (where the treatment condition of the participants in an experiment is not known to the observer), standardized instructions (e.g. to instruct all users of a questionnaire in the same way) and the use of physiological measures, such as pulse rate or body temperature.

Demand characteristics

Participants in investigations think about what it is they are doing, and may work out the researcher's aims. This is a problem as it can alter their behaviour, encouraging them to be 'good participants' and produce the results they think the researcher is expecting, or the opposite. The 'cues' or clues in the investigation, which help the participants to work out the aim, are called demand characteristics, and researchers try to keep these to a minimum. We will consider two ways that this can be done later in this book.

Experimenter bias

Researchers themselves may be a source of error in investigations. Think about how the researcher's own beliefs and expectations may affect their behaviour. Experimenters conduct research in the belief that there will be a difference in the outcome for participants in different conditions. This expectation might cause them to treat the participants differently, creating another source of influence on the participants other than the factor they are studying. This can be solved either by using 'standardized instructions', so that every participant is dealt with in exactly the same way, or by having an individual, who isn't aware of the aims of the study, in direct contact with the participants. In addition, when a researcher collects data, they might behave differently to people in each group. Again, this may be solved by using a naïve individual to collect the data or by asking the participants to self-report their responses.

What makes an ethically good study?

The use of human participants in psychological research has the potential to cause harm to participants and to be detrimental to the public face of psychology. To avoid these potential problems, psychologists follow ethical guidelines. In the UK, this advice is published by the British Psychological Society. Their guidelines raise the following key issues.

Deception

Participants should not be misled about the purpose of the study or the tasks it will involve. Sometimes, however, in order to ensure that participants do not work out the objective of the study, and alter their behaviour as a consequence, it may be essential to deceive them. In this case, after appropriate consultation with an ethical committee, researchers may find ways to reduce the potential problems arising from deception. One such way is to ask a similar group of people whether they would object to being deceived in this way and by telling the participants exactly what the purpose was after they have completed the study and inviting them to remove their results.

Informed consent

A full explanation of what the study will entail should be given to participants so that they can decide whether they want to take part.

Privacy and confidentiality

Participants have an entitlement to privacy, which concerns access to information that they would expect to be unavailable to others. This might include asking too deeply about their personal beliefs or memories, or observing them other than in public places where they expect to be seen.

Protection from harm

Procedures in studies should protect the participants, so they are at no greater risk of physical or psychological damage than they would be in their everyday life.

Independent variable
The factor which the researcher manipulates in an experiment to create different 'conditions' or 'levels' (to see its effect on the DV)

Right to withdraw

At the beginning of a study, participants should be made aware that they are entitled to leave at any point, regardless of any payment.

Debriefing

At the end of the study, researchers should ensure that participants are thanked and, where necessary, returned to their previous content state of mind.

Dependent variable
The factor which the researcher measures in an experiment (to see the effect of the IV)

What research methods do psychologists use?

Experiments

An experiment is an investigation that investigates the effect of one variable, called the independent variable, on another, called the dependent variable. This cause and effect relationship is explored in a controlled environment, to be certain that no factors other than the independent variable (IV) are causing changes in the dependent variable (DV).

Many of the studies you will read about in the text are experiments. Each has an independent and dependent variable. In addition, each has an **experimental design**, indicating how the IV was represented in different 'levels' or 'conditions' and a technique for measuring the DV.

The experimental design is the way the participants are allocated to conditions of the IV. There are different ways of achieving this including:

- *independent groups design* in which different participants are used in each level of the IV

- *repeated measured design* in which the same participants are used in every level of the IV.

Each design has advantages and disadvantages. In an independent groups design, there is a risk that the different groups of participants differ in some fundamental way. This might mean that any effect discovered in the outcome, i.e. any differences in the measures of the DV between groups, might be due to some underlying difference between the groups rather than the influence of the variable being manipulated. In a repeated measures design the participants are tested twice, so see the experimental situation twice. This is a disadvantage as the first exposure may affect their behaviour on the second occasion. For example, the participant may get better on a test with practice, or get bored and do worse.

Correlations

Experiments can be used when the variable to be studied can be manipulated, but sometimes this isn't possible. In situations when two potentially linked variables cannot be manipulated but can be measured over a range of values, we can look for a relationship between them. Such a relationship would be a **correlation**. The findings of correlational analyses can only tell us if two variables are linked, not whether the change in one is dependent on the change in the other, i.e. we cannot draw conclusions about cause and effect.

When the results of correlational analysis show that the two variables are related, this pattern will be one of two kinds, a positive or a negative correlation. In a **positive correlation**, the two variables increase together – as one increases, so does the other. In a **negative correlation**, as one variable increases the other decreases. Both are correlations. If there is no correlation, then participants with high scores on one variable will not consistently have either high or low scores on the other, but a mixture.

Self-report

Self-reports may be open-ended descriptions, such as patient diaries, or the data may be gathered in more structured ways, by asking

Experimental design
The arrangement for using the same or different participants in the conditions of an experiment

Correlation
A relationship between two variables

Positive correlation
A relationship between two variables such that they change together (as one increases, so does the other)

Negative correlation
A relationship between two variables such that as one variable increases the other decreases

predominantly closed questions, such as rating scales for the patient. Questionnaires (questions on paper or via the Internet) and interviews (face-to-face) both generate self-report data. Either can use open questions or closed ones. Interviews may be highly structured, like a spoken questionnaire, or may be more open, such as are used in unstructured interviews. The latter tend to be very subjective and it is difficult to determine whether they are valid or reliable, so questionnaires are often used in research.

Observations

When researchers want to study a particular behaviour, such as mobility or sociability, they use observations. These provide direct information about what the participant is actually doing in contrast to the indirect information that can be obtained through self-reports (and might be affected by bias or lying). To investigate the mobility of a patient with a painful chronic condition or the sociability of a bereaved person who does not seem to be overcoming their grief, observations could provide objective measures of the individual's quality of life.

Observations can be conducted directly or using recording systems such as CCTV or video. In all cases, ethical issues of privacy and consent must be considered. In order to conduct observations, researchers typically define a set of behaviours they intend to measure and use strategies, such as check lists to record them.

How are the findings of studies assessed?

Statistics are not designed to confuse you! They are there to simplify the mass of data produced by a study so that you can see at a glance what the findings show. This can be done in one of two basic ways, as descriptions or as interpretations. Descriptions can be visual, such as graphs, or numerical, such as averages. These are called descriptive statistics. Interpretations can be content based, such as when key themes are extracted from spoken interactions or texts, or can be mathematical inferences from numerical data. The latter are called inferential statistics. You will encounter different kinds of statistics both in the results of studies reported in this text and in your work. It is not essential for you to be able to name, choose or conduct inferential statistics but it is important that you understand their overall purpose, and that you have a sound grasp of descriptive statistics.

Descriptive statistics

When you encounter a group of numbers (called the 'data set'), such as a patient's temperature record, you are unlikely to look at every single piece of data. Instead you want to know about some overall patterns: What has their temperature been like in general? Has it been particularly low, or especially high? These are the questions that descriptive statistics answer.

Measures of central tendency

To describe a patient's typical temperature over a period of time, we want to know the 'average'. This is a measure of 'central tendency', i.e. a description of the 'middle' of the data and there are several different ways to work this out. The simplest is the mode. This is the number that appears most frequently in the data set, i.e. whatever temperature reading was most common in that record. Another way to work out the typical temperature would be to put all of the values in sequence from biggest to smallest and find the one in the middle of the data set. This is called the median (if there is an even number of temperature scores, you would add the two middle ones together and divide by two). The measure of central tendency you are most likely to encounter is the mean (or 'average'). This would be worked out by adding all the temperature figures together and dividing by the number of figures there are. For example, if a patient's temperature is taken three times a day for a week, there would be 21 figures. You would add all of the temperatures together, then divide by 21, to find the mean.

Measures of spread

Another piece of information you might want to know about your patient is the highest and lowest temperatures recorded. This is the range, the simplest measure of spread or 'dispersion'. It is sometimes written simply as the largest and smallest figures or, alternatively, the lowest score may be taken away from the highest to give a single figure.

There are other ways to express this spread of data, which are calculated in different ways. One you might encounter is called the standard deviation. This is also a single figure, and gives an indication of how spread out a data set is around the mean. When the data are very dispersed (many scores are widely spread) this produces a larger value for the standard deviation than when figures in the data set are more tightly clustered around the mean. So, a patient with a steady temperature would have a smaller standard deviation than one with a widely fluctuating temperature.

Graphs and charts

It is sometimes easier to see key information or a pattern in a data set when the results are presented visually. There are several different ways to do this, each of which is used for different reasons. Most graphs are drawn on two axes (lines at right angles which represent two variables) that meet in the bottom left-hand corner, at the 'origin'. The axis that goes horizontally across the bottom of the graph is called the x-axis and the vertical one up the side is called the y-axis (you can remember this with the hint: 'X is a-cross').

A bar chart is used to display data that are in separate categories and are not related to each other on a scale. A simple example might be a two-column chart of the success of a new health technique compared to an old one (see Figure 1.1). You are also likely to see more complex bar charts, such as paired bar charts, which show two comparative figures in each condition (see Figure 1.2).

Mode
A measure of central tendency or 'average': the most frequent score in a data set

Median
A measure of central tendency or 'average': the middle score in a data set when they are put in order from smallest to largest

Mean (Arithmetic mean)
A measure of central tendency or 'average': calculated by adding together all the scores in a data set and dividing by the number of scores

Range
A measure of spread or dispersion: quoted as either the largest and smallest scores in a data set or as the difference between these two

Bar chart
Graph with bars to represent values in separate categories

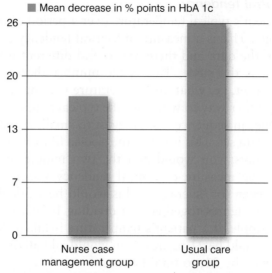

Figure 1.1   A bar chart showing the difference in reduction in blood glucose on diabetics after usual care or new-style care through nurse case management (Aubert *et al.*, 1998).

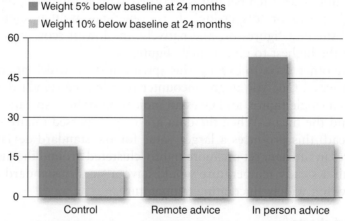

Figure 1.2   A paired bar chart that shows the number of people who have lost weight 5 per cent and 10 per cent below the baseline when given advice remotely and in person compared to no advice.

Histogram
Graph with bars to represent values in categories that are related to each other on a scale

A similar graph is a **histogram**, which also has bars but there are no gaps between them. The reason for this is because a histogram displays results that come from a continuous scale. The points along the x-axis are not just named categories or unconnected values. Instead, they represent measurements from an increasing sequence on which each point is directly related to the value of the previous one. The values up the y-axis are typically frequencies so the resulting graph, a frequency histogram, would show the number of data points of each value (or in each range of values) on the scale. The example in Figure 1.3 shows some data relating the percentage of the adult population who are obese (on the y-axis) to the continuous variable of time (on the x-axis).

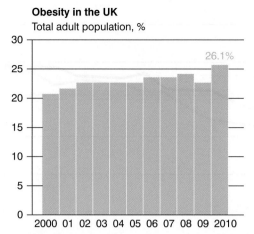

Obesity in the UK
Total adult population, %

Figure 1.3 Histogram showing the change in adult obesity in the UK, 2000–2010.

In a line graph both axes have continuous scales (although these may be grouped). Points are plotted as corresponding values on each scale, and then joined with a line, or a 'line of best fit', i.e. one which represents the general trend of the data. A line graph can be used in many ways, for example as an alternative to a histogram to show frequencies in values along a scale (**Figure 1.5** illustrates similar data to **Figure 1.3**). Alternatively, the results of an experiment with several continuous levels of the independent variable may be plotted on a histogram.

Line graph
Chart where both axes have continuous scales (although these may be grouped). Points are plotted as corresponding values on each scale, and then joined with a line, or a 'line of best fit', i.e. one that represents the general trend of the data.

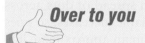

Over to you

What does the histogram in Figure 1.4 show?

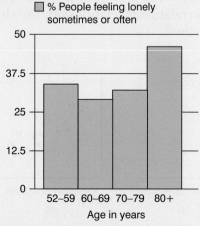

Figure 1.4 Histogram of loneliness in older adults (Beaumont, 2013)

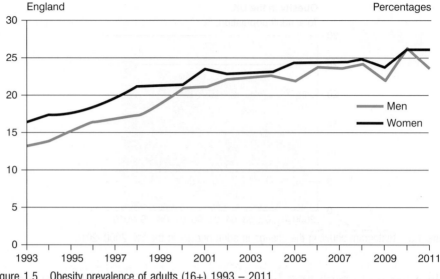

Figure 1.5   Obesity prevalence of adults (16+) 1993 – 2011

Scattergraph
Chart which
illustrates the
findings of a
correlational analysis,
showing a single dot
for the two scores
from each participant

A **scattergraph** is a way to represent correlational data. In a scattergraph, each dot or cross represents one individual's score on two variables. For example, a psychologist might use a scattergraph to show how older adults' cognitive ability, measured as their score on the recall of a word list, was related to their physical activity, as measured by the time per day that they spent walking. Figure 1.6 shows three examples of scattergraphs, with patterns of dots illustrating different relationships. Where there is no relationship between two variables, there will be an even spread of dots across the scattergraph. In a positive correlation, as one variable increases, so does the other. In a graph of this relationship, the dots lie in an approximate line rising out from the origin (i.e. sloping up to the right). In a negative correlation, as one variables rises the other falls. Here, the points form a 'line' sloping the other way (down from left to right). In both cases, the stronger the correlational relationship, the closer the dots are clustered to the imaginary 'line'.

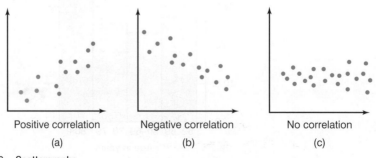

Positive correlation	Negative correlation	No correlation
(a)	(b)	(c)

Figure 1.6   Scattergraphs

Inferential statistics

When you look at a table or a graph of a set of data you can often see an obvious pattern – you can then be fairly sure that the results 'show something'. Sometimes, however, you might think that the difference between conditions, or the apparent correlation, is quite small. Researchers must ask the question *Is the pattern important enough to matter?* This measure of importance, or *significance*, can be judged mathematically. To decide whether a difference between conditions in an experiment, or a relationship in a correlational analysis, is significant calculations called inferential statistics are used. These 'statistical tests' judge whether it is probable that the pattern could have arisen just by chance. If this is (sufficiently) unlikely, they conclude that the pattern in the results is significant. You do not need to know about the statistical tests themselves, or how they are calculated. However, it is helpful to know that results of studies may, for example, be 'significant at $p \leq 0.05$'. This means that it is unlikely that the findings are simply due to chance, i.e. that it is probable (but not certain) that the effect they have found is a real one.

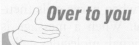 **Over to you**

Consider a set of data with a lot of individual numbers, such as the records of a person's pulse rate taken frequently over several days. What kind of statistical information would tell you about their typical pulse over the entire record?

What kind of statistical information would tell you about the variation in their pulse over the period?

If you wanted to look for a change in their pulse, perhaps before compared to after a procedure, what kind of statistical information might be helpful?

If you read that there was 'a statistically significant reduction in blood pressure' for patients given a particular drug, what would you conclude, and how sure would you be about your conclusion?

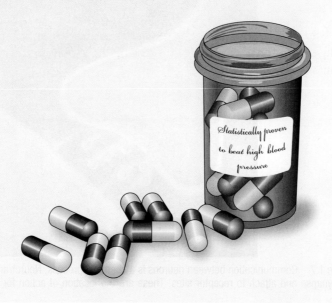

THE BRAIN, THE NERVOUS SYSTEM AND THE ENDOCRINE SYSTEM

You may recall from the beginning of this chapter that the biological basis of the nervous system was important in the early roots of psychology, and is still a key feature of psychology today.

Psychologists are interested in both the structure and the function of the nervous system. The overall structure can be divided into the central nervous system (the brain and spinal cord) and the peripheral nervous system (the nerve cells in the rest of the body). Within the brain, many different areas and structures have been identified, through studying dissected brains of humans and animals and, more recently, with brain scans. The peripheral nervous system includes the somatic nerves and the nerves of the autonomic nervous system. The somatic nerves include motor nerves, carrying information out from the brain for movement, and sensory nerves, which carry information inwards from the body to the brain, for example about touch and pain. The autonomic nervous system operates unconsciously, and controls functions such as digestion and the production of hormones.

The nervous system is built up of individual nerve cells called neurons. These send electrical messages along their length but when nerve cells (neurons) interact, the activity that occurs is **biochemical**. When a message is passed from one neuron to the next it is a chemical signal: molecules called neurotransmitters are released from one neuron, travel across the gap between the cells (the synapse) and attach to specific locations (receptor sites) on the membrane of the next neuron. This causes the message to be continued along the next neuron (see Figure 1.7).

Biochemical
Relating to the chemistry of living things, such as the human body

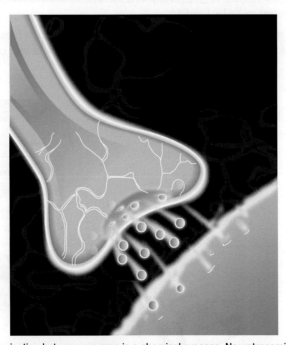

Figure 1.7   Communication between neurons is a chemical process. Neurotransmitter molecules cross the synapse and attach to receptor sites. These are the location of action for many drugs.

There are several different kinds of neurons. Receptor cells, or nerve endings, detect stimuli, such as light in the eye or pain all over the body. Neurons with the central nervous system, called interneurons, are very short and make many, many synapses with other neurons to form a network. Outside the central nervous system, in the body, further neurons can be found some, (but not all) of which, are surrounded by an insulating fatty layer (called a myelin sheath), which helps them to conduct electrical impulses quickly. One type of nerve fibre carrying information about pain (the A-delta fibres) are myelinated, so can send information about peripheral tissue damage back to the brain very quickly.

The nervous system provides the body's 'rapid response' system but we also have a communication system that provides a slower, more sustained response. This is called the endocrine system. Hormones, chemicals released from glands into the blood, target specific organs and tissues (including other glands). They influence the biochemistry of their target, producing changes in functioning. One important example of the role of hormones in psychological processes is the response to stress. In response to a sudden stressor, our nervous system reacts quickly and then we release the hormone adrenalin to sustain our reaction.

FREUD AND DEFENCE MECHANISMS

Freud's work on the unconscious, the personality and on understanding and overcoming mental illnesses has been enormously influential. Freud believed that much of our mind, and the motives, memories, fears and desires within it, are unconscious; we are unaware of its contents. Nevertheless, these unconscious thoughts could affect us in many ways, for instance by motivating our behaviour (which could therefore be surprising to us) and by producing the symptoms of mental illness.

A key idea that you will encounter in several chapters is that of defence mechanisms. These are unconscious strategies that help to protect our conscious (or aware mind) from unpleasant thoughts and feelings. Freud proposed many different defence mechanisms, including denial and repression. In denial, we can unconsciously refuse to admit an unpleasant fact to ourselves. We may deny that we need to stop a damaging behaviour, such as excessive drinking, in order to protect our health. Repression operates to protect our conscious mind by preventing us from retrieving unpleasant memories, so we cannot dwell on them or worry about them. A patient who has been recently bereaved may repress the memory of their loved one's death, so that they do not have to accept that they will never return.

LEARNING THEORIES

The behaviourists and subsequent researchers, studying how we acquire new behaviours, have proposed several different explanations. These are used to explain many different aspects of health behaviour throughout the text.

Conditioning

Two types of conditioning were described and explained by the early behaviourists: classical conditioning by Pavlov and operant conditioning by Thorndike and Skinner.

Classical conditioning

Classical conditioning suggests that we learn associations between a 'new' situation (the neutral stimulus) and an 'old' one (the unconditioned stimulus) to which the individual already exhibits a behaviour (the unconditioned response). Repeated pairings of the neutral stimulus and unconditioned stimulus result in the generation of a behaviour resembling the unconditioned response when presented with the neutral stimulus. Once this association has been established, the neutral stimulus is called the conditioned stimulus and the resulting response the conditioned response.

This theory can explain why a dog salivates when it sees a tin of food before it has even been opened. The tin and the food are associated in time so eventually even the tin, in the absence of any food, can cause salivation. Such classically conditioned associations could also account for the placebo effect (see below).

Classical conditioning

Dog food → Salivation
Dog food + dog food tin → Salivation
Dog food tin → Salivation

Pain of injection → Fear
Pain of injection + seeing needle → Fear
Needle → Fear

Taking (real) tablets → Pain reduction (due to tablets)
Seeing and taking tablets → Pain reduction (due to tablets)
Seeing and taking (placebo) tablets → Pain reduction (due to conditioning)

Operant conditioning

In operant conditioning, behaviours that are followed by pleasant consequences (reinforcers) are performed more often, those with unpleasant consequence (punishers) less often. Reinforcers are always nice and always increase the frequency of the behaviours they follow but they may be positive reinforcers (nice when they happen) or negative reinforcers (nice when they stop). An example of a positive reinforcer is the use of badges and stickers. Blood donors can be rewarded for their effort by giving them badges, children can be reinforced for co-operative behaviour in a clinic with a smiley sticker. These reinforcers increase the probability that a donor will return next time or that a child will co-operate again. Taking painkillers acts as a negative reinforcer. The pain is unpleasant, if taking medication makes the pain go away, the patient is more likely to take the medication again next time.

Social learning theory

This theory explains the effect of a model on the behaviour of an observer. When an individual (the learner) sees another person (the model) performing a behaviour, they are likely to imitate them. This is social learning. The learner is more likely to imitate the behaviour if the model is the same gender, has high status and is likeable. They are also more likely to do so if they see the model themselves being rewarded for the action. For example, if a parent responds to an injection by wincing, the child may do so too. In contrast, if one child is praised for letting a nurse change a dressing without a fuss, another child is more likely to copy the good behaviour than if the model was not praised.

THEORIES FROM COGNITIVE PSYCHOLOGY

The cognitive approach is based on the idea that we process information. This means that theories about taking in, using and retrieving information are all the domain of cognitive psychology. You will encounter cognitive theories relating to perception, memory and to other aspects of the way that we interpret information about health.

The locus of control

Rotter (1966) described the concept of locus of control, a measure that describes the extent to which an individual perceives that they themselves or some other, external force, is responsible for determining the course of events in their lives. The idea has been applied both to health and pain, using the health locus of control (Wallston *et al.*, 1978) and the pain locus of control (Manning and Wright, 1983). These measures assess the level of self-determination versus external causation an individual perceives with respect to their health or experience of pain. Essentially, it suggests that patients who attribute control to factors they cannot govern, such as luck or whether they have a good consultant, are described as having an external locus of control. Those who believe that they are responsible for actions that affect themselves, such as remembering to take their medication regularly, have an internal locus of control. So an individual's locus of control can clearly affect how actively they engage in their own pain management. In addition, it appears to have a bearing on their actual experience of pain.

Coping strategies

Another patient characteristic is the idea of coping strategies, i.e. the extent to which the individual employs emotion- or problem-focused strategies for dealing with difficulties. Where there are useful steps the patient can take to deal with their own pain, problem-focused strategies are beneficial. For example, when a patient adheres to the advised schedule of exercise, rest or painkillers and this successfully limits their pain, they gain from being problem-focused. However, where there is little or nothing patients can do to minimize their suffering, as when an injured patient is awaiting surgery, emotion-focused strategies that allow them to ignore the problem or blame someone else will be more helpful.

KEY POINTS

- Psychology is a diverse subject with a range of different approaches, which look at the process of the mind and behaviour in different ways.

- Psychologists use a range of different methods in their research and most of these are scientific. They also aim to ensure that their research is ethical.

- Physiological psychology considers the extent to which the biological processes of the nervous system and hormones can explain psychological phenomena.

- Psychodynamic psychology explores the influence of the unconscious on our thinking and behaviour.

- Behaviourism focuses on observable behaviour and uses the findings to explain phenomena in terms of stimuli and responses, rewards and punishments.

- Cognitive psychologists investigate the way we process information, looking at functions such as memory and factors that affect it.

CONCLUSIONS

Psychology is a relatively new science so, unlike subjects such as chemistry, it does not have a single underlying principle used to explain all the phenomena it encompasses. There have been many approaches to psychology over time, and most are still influential in our current understanding. Psychologists in all the domains make observations, propose theories to explain them and use a range of different research methods in studies to test their theories. The findings of this research are often analyzed statistically, using both descriptive and inferential statistics.

RAPID RECAP

1 What is the difference between a behaviourist explanation and a cognitive one?

2 What did Freud suggest could control our behaviour that made his explanations different from other theories?

3 Why do psychologists use statistics in their research?

If you have difficulty with any of the questions, read through the section again to refresh your understanding before moving on.

KEY REFERENCES

Other references are listed on the supporting website.

Aubert, R.E., Herman, W.H., Waters, J., Moore, W., Sutton, D., Peterson, B.L., Bailey, C.M. and Koplan, J.P. (1998) Nurse case management to improve glycemic control in diabetic patients in a health maintenance organization. A randomized, controlled trial. *Annals of Internal Medicine*, 129 (8): 605–12.

Beaumont, J. (2013) Measuring national well-being – older people and loneliness. Office for National Statistics, 11 April 2013.

Health and Social Care Information Centre (2013) Statistics on Obesity, Physical activity and diet: England. HSCI, 20th February, 2013.

CHAPTER 2

COMMUNICATION IN THE HEALTH AND SOCIAL CARE SETTING

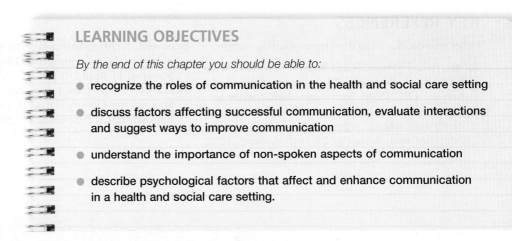

LEARNING OBJECTIVES

By the end of this chapter you should be able to:

- recognize the roles of communication in the health and social care setting

- discuss factors affecting successful communication, evaluate interactions and suggest ways to improve communication

- understand the importance of non-spoken aspects of communication

- describe psychological factors that affect and enhance communication in a health and social care setting.

I n this chapter we explore psychological factors relating to communication. Some are common to all settings, such as the value of listening as well as speaking. In other ways the health and social care setting is special. Patients may not communicate readily and adhering to normal conventions, such as avoiding the invasion of personal space, may not be practically possible. Such issues make effective communication very valuable.

Even though nurses are constantly engaged with patients, sometimes their communication skills are not sufficient to meet patient needs (Macleod Clark, 1982). We will consider a range of factors in interactions with the aim of helping you to understand and to evaluate the impact of your own communication at work and to improve it.

Communication
A two-way process of interaction that is dependent on the reception of, and feedback in response to, information

WHAT IS COMMUNICATION?

Insel and Roth (1996, p. 86) define communication as 'the process by which we establish contact and exchange information with others'. This simple definition draws attention to many of the key issues in communication:

- Communication can only be effective if we have established contact – our audience must be paying attention or we will simply be ignored.
- Communication is a process – it is not a single, simple act.
- Communication requires an exchange – it is a two-way event.

In a busy ward environment, or when dealing with patients whose communication skills are impaired, it is important to make certain that the receiver, the person for whom the message is intended, is going to see or hear the communication initiated by the sender and that they will recognize that it is meant for them.

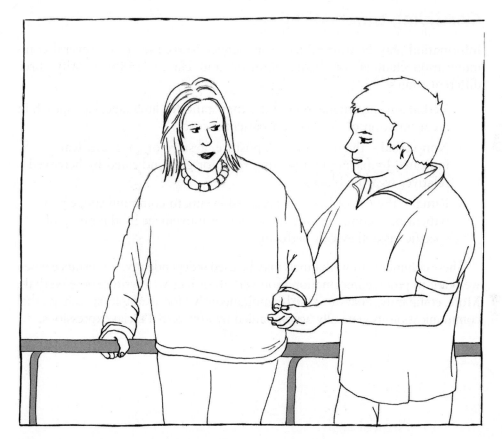

Which communication channels can you see here? And what functions do they serve?

The communication cycle

Communication is an interactive process. In the communication cycle, Figure 2.1, the sender emits a message and a response is produced by the receiver (feedback), which is received by the initial sender. Each stage has potential for error. Is the message encoded clearly by the sender? Does it reach the receiver? Is it understood by the receiver?

To identify and meet a patient's needs, health and social care staff need to be sure that the answer to each of these questions is 'yes'. This can be determined from the patient's feedback.

Communication cycle
An interactive process between communicators that consists of messages being sent, received and responded to with feedback to the orginator of the message

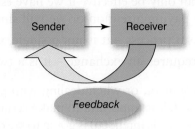

Figure 2.1   The communication cycle

Classifying communication

Information may be transmitted from sender to receiver using several communication channels or media. Stratton and Hayes (1988) identify three different routes:

- **Verbal** – using language or codes that stand for language, e.g. speech in a consultation or symbols on patient records.
- **Non-verbal** – the use of dress, posture, gesture or gaze, e.g. fear indicated by pacing in a waiting room or grief indicated by bereaved relatives wearing black.
- **Ritual** – the use of highly structured events to communicate, e.g. a patient may communicate their level of movement by the range of specific tasks they can perform.

These communication channels may be used independently, for instance when we point to provide information (non-verbal) or receive a written note (verbal). More commonly, they are used simultaneously, for example speech (verbal communication) is generally accompanied by non-verbal facial expressions.

Student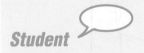

Student nurse on a surgical ward

Communication and caring – the importance of explanations to patients
'Last week a patient was checked in and he had signed a consent form for a TURP*. I went over to him to help him get washed the next day, after the operation. He said "Oh, I didn't realize that they would put a tube in there, and I didn't realize I'd have a drip. I thought they were going to cut me". I said, "Well did the doctor not explain to you when you were admitted?", and he said that if he had, he had not taken it in. I said, "Did you sign a consent form?" "Oh yes", he said.

I think this happens quite frequently, probably because people are so nervous about having an operation, and perhaps they are too in awe of the consultant to ask any questions. So really it is important that informed consent is signed for after careful explanation and checking of understanding.'

*TURP Transurethral prostatectomy – removal of the prostate using the same urethral route as for urinary catheter insertion.

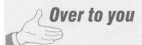

Over to you

Identify the medium for communication used in each of the following examples:

● Diagnostic radiographer wearing a formal badge to indicate their status and role to patients.

● A patient communicating their concerns by saying how they feel about having a general anaesthetic.

● A student on placement signalling that they need help with a drip by making eye contact with a qualified practitioner.

Reflective activity

Try to create a list of examples of communication being used for different functions in health and social care settings. Can you identify for each situation:

● The sender(s) and receiver(s)?

● Whether the situation is formal or informal?

● Whether the communication is predominantly verbal, non-verbal, ritual or mixed?

● In each case, consider the purpose of the interaction for each sender and receiver.

In your list you probably found a wide range of functions for communication. These functions can be divided into two broad categories:

● **Informational communication** – to transmit facts from one individual to another, e.g. when patients tell nurses that they are in pain or when a radiographer shows a patient how they need to position themselves for an X-ray.

● **Supportive communication** – to provide understanding, sympathy, reassurance or encouragement to patients, e.g. in the face of terminal diagnoses, unpleasant treatment or bereavement.

Hall *et al.* (1988) identified these two key goals in a medical encounter, describing them as 'instrumental tasks' (e.g. asking and answering questions) and 'socio-emotional tasks' (e.g. social conversation and partnership building). Much of the communication in health and social care falls into the former category, despite evidence that the role of supportive communication is both important and neglected. Teutsch (2003) observed that simply giving the patient the opportunity to air their concerns to a caring professional will have a therapeutic benefit.

Reflective activity

www.patient.co.uk is a website offering patients the opportunity to discuss their experiences, e.g. of treatment and support, with fellow sufferers. The role played by supportive communication from such websites, however, raises issues:

- How might the anonymity of the Internet assist communication for some patients?
- For what reasons might the provision of information be important for patients?
- Why should we be cautious about encouraging patients to use websites?

Communication failures

Communication failures can arise with either informational or supportive functions. Practitioners and patients (or practitioners differing in status or discipline) enter into interactions with different aims. Medically, communication serves to diagnose and treat a biological pathology, i.e. is informational. For the patient, communication needs may be personal, such as for reassurance. This difference in function may account for misdiagnosis (through lack of information from patients) and dissatisfied patients (lack of support from health and social carers). Neither communicator has fully achieved their goal because their intentions at the outset were different. As patients typically perceive their health and social carers to be higher in status this means they are less likely to feed back with queries or to check the information they receive.

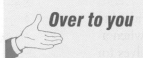

Over to you

Communication failure can arise from a breakdown at any point in the communication cycle. Identify the point at which the cycle is broken in each of these instances:

- A midwife mumbles when she asks a mother in the midst of labour, a question.
- A patient refuses to respond when prompted to express his anxieties about an operation.
- A student's reply to a question about a patient during a ward handover is interrupted by a contribution from another member of staff.
- A patient cannot hear a question being asked by her social worker about her recent domestic abuse problems.

Now think of two more scenarios in which communication breaks down.

KEY POINTS

● Seek feedback to be sure your message has been received and understood.

● Remember that the patient's reason for communicating may be different from yours but no less important.

WHY DO WE NEED TO COMMUNICATE IN HEALTH AND SOCIAL CARE SETTINGS?

The Fifth Principle of Nursing Practice, Principle E says:

> *'Nurses and nursing staff are at the heart of the communication process: they assess, record and report on treatment and care, handle information sensitively and confidentially, deal with complaints effectively, and are conscientious in reporting the things they are concerned about.'*

An NHS study of patient deterioration (Luettel *et al.*, 2007) concluded that communication issues were the main problem area in incidents involving avoidable deterioration in patient condition. The report identified that staff may not adequately inform each other regarding patients' care, especially during handovers and transfers. When there is a lot of information to exchange, and especially where it is hard for inexperienced staff to understand, it may be too much and difficult to remember.

Psychological research has identified specific aspects of communication, which act as barriers, such as interruptions; or help to overcome the barriers, for example the use of questions. As we will see later on, patients' recall of the information they have been given affects their compliance with advice. In a **meta-analysis**, Haskard-Zolnierek and DiMatteo (2009) found that patient adherence to treatment regimes was poor when these are communicated poorly but training in communication skills improved this.

Many aspects of communication have been shown to affect health-related interactions (Table 2.1).

In a patient satisfaction survey about nursing and patient/visitor communication in an emergency department, over 80 per cent of patients were very satisfied in relation to their important communication needs (Pytel *et al.*, 2009). This satisfaction was largely shared by the health and social care professionals, which is important as service providers must recognize what aspects matter to patients so they can meet their communication needs. McCabe (2004) also found that health and social care professionals could communicate well with patients, for example demonstrating attention, empathy and being friendly, but that to do so they needed a patient-centred model of communication whereas most hospital health and social care requires a task-centred approach.

Meta-analysis
A technique for investigating data from many different but related studies in which the data are combined to produce an overall estimate of the findings

Table 2.1 Communication factors associated with positive outcomes (Beck *et al.*, 2002)	
Verbal behaviours	**Non-verbal behaviours**
Empathy	Head nodding
Reassurance	Leaning forwards
Patient-centred questioning styles	Turning the body towards the patient
History taking	Uncrossed legs and arms
Explanations	Less mutual gaze
Positive reinforcement	
Humour	
Information sharing	
Friendliness	
Courtesy	
Summarizing and clarification	

KEY POINTS

● Poor communication can lead to patient deterioration (e.g. during handovers and transfers) and staff misunderstandings (especially for inexperienced colleagues).

● A huge range of verbal and non-verbal strategies help in communication and training in such skills can help to overcome communication problems.

● Nurses typically communicate well with patients but the patients' needs often conflict with the task-oriented needs of the nurse.

COMMUNICATION STYLES

Many communication models discriminate between doctor-centred and patient-centred styles (Table 2.2). They were formulated in the context of general practice, so focus on interactions between doctors and patients and on short consultations. Nevertheless they offer a useful insight into nurse-patient communication.

A doctor-centred style concentrates on the practitioner asking the patient questions to obtain information about their medical condition and providing them with advice as a result. The 'communication' is two-way but is directed by one of the participants. Berry *et al.* (2003) found that, in 55 per cent of consultations with cancer patients, clinicians interrupted when the patient was trying to provide information or ask a question.

In contrast, a patient-centred approach aims to ensure that the patient is treated as an individual rather than a commodity. The patient is active, asking and answering questions and responding to requests with opinions as well as facts.

Table 2.2 Different communication styles seen in practitioner-patient interactions		
	Doctor-centred	**Patient-centred**
Focus of doctor	His or her own status and control of the situation	To identify the patient's needs and adjust his or her own activities to satisfy both individuals
Actions of doctor	<ul><li>Gathers information</li><li>Asks direct, closed and rhetorical (self-answering) questions</li><li>Asks about medical 'facts'</li><li>Decides on outcome for patient and instructs them</li></ul>	<ul><li>Listens and considers what the patient is saying</li><li>Observes and encourages patient to express themselves</li><li>Asks about patient's ideas and for clarification, indicates understanding</li><li>Involves patient in decision-making</li></ul>
Expectations of patient	<ul><li>Passivity</li><li>Asks few questions</li><li>Does not influence the consultation</li></ul>	<ul><li>Active engagement</li><li>Asks questions</li><li>Influences the consultation</li></ul>

Patient-centred consultations are more likely to enable the patients to influence the outcome and are generally preferred by patients. Langewitz *et al.* (2010) investigated the effect of a communication skills training programme for oncology nurses. They found that many aspects of communication improved and particularly that the nurses displayed more empathetic responses to patients' emotional cues and the patients were able to speak for longer without being interrupted.

It might be assumed that all patients would prefer a consultative (patient-led) approach but some patients, including those under great stress or who are very ill, like the confident, directive style of doctor-led encounters. Others may not want to be involved in decision-making. For example, Blanchard *et al.* (1988) found that, although most wanted information, only two-thirds of cancer patients wished to participate in decisions about their own treatment. Here, the reassurance offered by the absolute opinions of professionals may be more important than the need to feel involved.

RESEARCH IN BRIEF

Brady (2009) Hospitalized children's view of a good nurse

Aim: To investigate five attributes of a nurse from a child's perspective: communication, professional competence, safety, professional appearance and virtues.

Procedure: 11 boys and 11 girls, (mean 10 years-old) were interviewed and asked to draw a picture of (or write or talk about) a good nurse and a bad nurse (without providing a definition of these). The content of these contributions was analyzed. The children were then interviewed further to check the interpretation of their drawings.

Findings: Communication was found to be a key component of the good nurse's attributes. For example, a good nurse used 'terms of endearment' when communicating, for example: '... she calls me sweetie pie. (John age 12)' (p. 548), which makes the child feel special. The children also liked praise for being brave: '... maybe, sometimes just to like tell 'em well done for being a good person because they've just had an injection or something and it really hurt. (Anna age 11)' (p. 548). The children were also aware of tone of voice and body language, for example noting that a good nurse didn't shout but used a 'nice', 'calm', 'cheerful' or 'kind' voice when speaking to them. Bad nurses in contrast were 'bad tempered', 'bossy', 'angry' or 'grumpy' and didn't listen to them. Interestingly, one 11 year-old described the importance of patience and politeness and showed an awareness of reciprocity between patients and staff: 'They're manners at the end of the day and you don't want to be rude to them otherwise they are gonna be rude to you and it causes violence and that's what the hospital doesn't want.'

Conclusion: In terms of communication, it is important, at least for children, that nurses treat them kindly and politely, offering at least some of the attributes of a good parent. (Note that this is in contrast to the way older patients prefer to be treated, as Woolhead *et al.* (2004) found that they saw overfamiliarity with patients as disrespectful.)

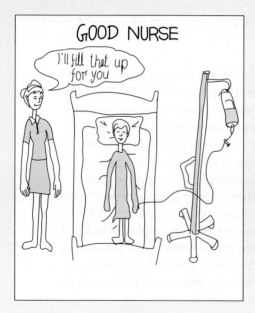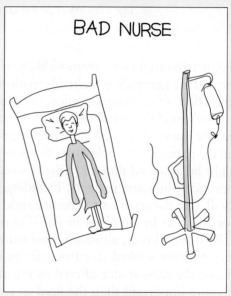

For Matthew (aged nine) a good nurse was one who came to change his empty intravenous fluid bag.

HEALTH PROFESSIONALS AS SKILLED COMMUNICATORS

The term 'bedside manner' and its positive or negative connotations suggest that there are good and not-so-good ways for health professionals and patients to communicate. It is important that health professionals are skilled communicators as they often deal with people in personal and physical circumstances that can interfere with effective communication. Patients may be:

- in unfamiliar surroundings
- interacting with people they do not know well, if at all
- nervous or anxious
- embarrassed
- in pain
- very tired or under the influence of sedative drugs
- unable to comprehend events, concepts or words that are used
- unwilling to ask questions.

All these factors are barriers to communication making effective interaction harder. For example, if patients are reluctant to ask questions, this makes the task of judging whether they understand more difficult. However, good patient care relies on an effective relationship between the patient and those working with them. Health and social care professionals need information from patients in order to perform their jobs effectively and ethically, to ensure rapid recovery, and to maximize the patient's comfort and dignity. In this section we will be looking at the skills that health and social care professionals need to employ for successful interactions in even the most difficult situations.

Caris-Verhallen *et al.* (2000) found that in the case of elderly-care health and social care, a training programme based on video analysis did allow health and social care professionals to provide patients with more information. The trained health and social care professionals used more open-ended questions and were rated to be more involved, warmer and less patronizing.

In recognition of the importance of the need for effective communication, the document 'Essence of Care (2010) Benchmarks for Communication' sets out the standards for nurses in relation to communication.

KEY POINTS

- A patient-centred style of communication, which empowers patients, is generally preferred.
- Patients are experiencing personal and physical distress, which interferes with communication.

SPOKEN COMMUNICATION
Speech

'Spoken communication' is used exclusively to refer to actual speech whereas 'verbal communication' can be used to mean any word-based communication, so also includes written messages, fingerspelling and Braille.

Fingerspelling
An alphabet formed by hand shapes used by people with hearing impairments to spell out single words

Braille
A form of printing in which letters of the alphabet are represented by patterns of raised dots. It is used by people with visual impairment to read (and produce) documents

Reflective activity

Emotions, for example fear, rage, misery, disbelief or being overwhelmed (with relief or pain), may affect our ability to communicate. These states can be triggered by our own ill - health, bereavement, our feelings for sick loved ones or our experiences with colleagues. The environment, such as being in an entirely unfamiliar situation, may also affect us, making us less competent communicators.

Think of instances in which you, a patient, a colleague or a visitor has been 'lost for words'. Under what circumstances did this arise? What reasons do you think might account for your examples? In these situations, what other cues tell us what a person means or how they feel?

Health and social care, like all professions, uses specialist terminology. You are learning new terms at the moment and will become fluent in the 'register' or language of health and social care. Being unfamiliar with the terms and shorthand that health and social carers use in their day-to-day speech disadvantages patients. When the register is misused, excluding the patient from the interaction, it is referred to as jargon. Hadlow and Pitts (1991) investigated knowledge of common medical terms. Although doctors understood 70 per cent, patients understood only 36 per cent. Patients are often reluctant to ask for clarification if they do not understand and may find this frightening or isolating. Williams *et al.* (2011) found that an important role of community matrons was to help patients to understand medical jargon, thus contributing to and enhancing their perceptions of their care.

Jargon
Inappropriate use of professional terminology that excludes individuals, such as the patient or their supporters, from the interaction

Some patients will be well versed in current terminology and feel insulted if medical staff 'dumb-down' their explanations, so judging each individually is important. In a study of effectiveness of discharge information given to patients, Giuse *et al.* (2012) measured patients' literacy. When tested on their understanding at the time, and 2 weeks later, those given information matched to their ability had better understanding than those given routine instructions.

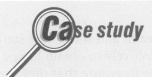

Case study

An inappropriate level of communication

A patient who was a well-qualified biologist and health and social care tutor at degree level reported her feelings following consultations in preparation for a laparoscopy and subsequent hysterectomy. After descriptions of 'periscopes in her tummy' once she had been 'popped under' and 'being pulled together like a draw-string bag' the female consultant gynaecologist had failed to inform or reassure her at all. After giving her the opportunity to ask questions, the level of her explanations didn't change despite the patient's obvious knowledge.

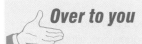

Reflective activity

What was the consultant attempting to do? Was she successful? What could she have done to improve her communication?

Over to you

As you are in training as a health professional, many of the terms that baffle patients will now be familiar to you. To enable you to imagine what it might be like for patients, consider how you would feel if you were told any of the following about a problem with your house:

- 'The A test was negative.' (Is that good or bad?)
- 'The B are creeping.' (Should they be?)
- 'We can detect some X but it's nothing to worry about.' (Isn't it?)

Would you feel safe?

The diversity of language means that it can also be ambiguous, that is, have two alternative meanings, leading to confusion. For example, how should a patient awaiting discharge have interpreted the comment 'You'll need to stay in' – in where? Was the intended meaning 'indoors once you get home' or 'in hospital'? Another example involved a deaf patient who didn't understand the written question 'Are you opening your bowels regularly?' He definitely hadn't opened anything so replied 'No' and was given daily doses of (quite unnecessary) laxative until he complained of diarrhoea.

Questions

In order to elicit vital information from patients, health and social care staff ask questions and need to take care to use these effectively to obtain honest, accurate and complete information. They also have to ensure that they are not distressing the patient. Depending on the nature of the information required, different questioning techniques are used.

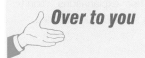

Barriers to communication

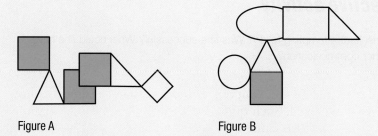

Figure A   Figure B

Try this exercise sitting back-to-back with a partner. Give them a sheet of paper and a pen and ask them to draw the shape you are going to describe. Warn them that they cannot look or ask questions, although they can say 'I don't understand'. Start by describing the layout of Figure A. When you think they have finished, repeat the exercise with Figure B, this time allowing them to ask any questions they like. Finally, both of you look at the originals and their drawings.

- How did the second drawing compare to the first? Why?
- What did it feel like to be the one trying to impart or to receive information?
- What implications does this have for health and social care settings?

Closed questions have a restricted range of possible answers, e.g. spoken questions, such as 'What is your name?' or 'Have you taken this medication before?' Closed questions on printed material, such as registration forms and other questionnaires, would include 'What is your date of birth' and 'Do you smoke?' Here, patients often select the most appropriate answer from a list (e.g. 'Do you take exercise? No/occasionally/daily').

An open question allows the patient freedom to provide longer, detailed answers. Such questions can elicit information about a patient's emotions, for example how they feel about their diagnosis or a forthcoming operation. In addition, they may provide access to important but unpredictable information that may not be obtained otherwise, helping staff to understand patients' needs more fully. Compare the two conversations in Box 2.1.

BOX 2.1

(A) **Nurse:** Hello, Mr Brown. You're feeling better aren't you?

Mr Brown: Yes, a bit.

Nurse: I'd like to take your drip out, are you ready for me to do it now you've finished your tea?

Mr Brown: Yes, OK.

(B) **Nurse:** Hello, Mr Brown. How are you feeling today?

Mr Brown: A bit queasy, I think I drank my tea too quickly.

Nurse: Your drip needs to come out, how do you feel about me doing it now?

Mr Brown: I'd rather you didn't – could you do it in a few minutes when I've settled down again?

1 Which conversation uses open questions and which closed questions?

2 Which conversation would lead to better patient care?

Berry *et al.* (2003) found that, in consultation with cancer patients, approximately 85 per cent of questions were closed and only 15 per cent were open questions.

The wording of a leading question implies, either directly or indirectly, that a particular answer is required. Such questions can result in misinformation from the patient. They can also cause changes in patient's memory of what was said. For example, a woman who is asked 'Would your preference be for a vaginal or abdominal hysterectomy?' would be contradicting the questioner if she volunteered the reply that she did not want a hysterectomy at all. Consider the conversations in Box 2.2.

> **Leading question**
> One in which information is presented that implies that a particular answer is required or expected

BOX 2.2

(A)

Surgeon: The operation went very well, are you gaining more feeling in your foot now?

Patient: Yes, a little.

Surgeon: Good, so we'll start you on physiotherapy tomorrow and we'll have you up and walking and ready to return home in no time. That'll be good, you're looking forward to getting back aren't you?

Patient: Yes.

(B)

Surgeon: Are you aware of any change in the amount you can feel in your foot yet?

Patient: Yes, I think there's a little more feeling.

Surgeon: Good, so we'll start you on physiotherapy tomorrow and we'll have you up and walking and ready to return home in no time. How do you feel about going home?

Patient: I'm keen to get home but worried about managing the stairs, as I still can't bend my ankle very well.

● Which conversation would provide more information about the patient's feelings and physical progress?

Listening

When we think of verbal communication our focus tends to fall on the role of speech but without listening, spoken words alone cannot complete the communication cycle as any 'feedback' would be unrelated to the initial message. Randall *et al.* (2008) found that child patients identified being willing to listen and good at it, as an important characteristic of a good health and social care professional.

It is common for speakers to use the time when they are not talking to decide what to say next – hence they are not listening to the reply. To become an effective listener, we need to pay attention to both the words and the non-verbal aspects of the sender's message (see next section). Effective listening is an important skill in counselling and Stickley (2011) has extended ideas from counselling to the nursing context. The following guide aims to help you to improve your own communication:

S – Sit at an angle to the client
U – Uncross legs and arms
R – Relax
E – Eye contact
T – Touch
Y – Your intuition

The acronym SURETY helps to recall these ideas but remember, these are only guidelines not inflexible rules. A very open posture (with uncrossed arms and legs) may imply that you are unprofessional, reducing the effectiveness of communication. Similarly, in personal discussion about symptoms or treatments, patients may be too embarrassed to make eye contact.

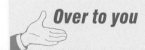

Over to you

The following messages might be attended to by a listener. Identify whether each of them are linguistic, paralinguistic or non-verbal:

- A patient, who is talking loudly and quickly, indicating that they are angry.

- A visitor, who is sitting beside a patient's bed with their arms folded and legs tucked in, looking very white, and who seems to be upset.

- A colleague, whose speech is punctuated with pauses, suggesting that they are anxious.

- A hospital receptionist, who says that she has booked an appointment for a patient.

Another concept from counselling is active listening: a way to encourage the client to explore their thoughts and feelings. Active listening can use the following techniques:

- **Mirroring** – reflecting back the client's words or postures to encourage expansion, e.g. to a client who says 'I feel rather empty', you might reply, 'Empty?'
- **Empathy-building statements** – indicating attention and an attempt to understand, e.g. 'I imagine that … .'
- **Silence** – to allow the client uninterrupted time to think.

Care must be taken to ensure that mirroring, whether verbal or postural, is not too overt, as this may appear sarcastic, and that rephrasing gives an accurate representation of feelings. This can be verified with simple questions such as 'It seems as though you are … is that right?' Mirroring is also seen in non-verbal communication although usually it is unconscious and seen as a sign of having developed a good rapport. We will consider such non-verbal aspects in the next section.

KEY POINTS

- Avoid jargon as it can confuse and exclude the patient: terms that are ordinary to you may be unfamiliar to them.
- Try to match your speech to each patient's level of understanding, to find a balance between risking being confusing or being patronizing.
- Be careful to avoid ambiguities, to ask open questions and to avoid leading questions to gain the maximum possible, and most accurate, information from patients.
- Try to listen to patients actively, and indicate that you understand them.

NON-VERBAL COMMUNICATION

Whilst words convey important information and opinions, and can ask questions, the non-verbal aspects of communication provide a context within which these messages are interpreted. These additional cues can subtly alter the meaning of the speech they accompany and allow a nurse to establish rapport with the patient.

Paralanguage: the non-verbal aspects of speech

Paralanguage encompasses all the ways that the voice is used to convey meaning, excluding the meaning of the words themselves. Using video analysis of consultation, Henry *et al.* (2011) found that both patients and doctors based judgements on non-verbal cues such as gestures, body language, eye contact and facial expression.

Try listening to some speech – a live show or an interview on a foreign language radio station. Even though you may have little idea of the content you will be able to identify some aspects of the way the speaker uses their voice. Paralinguistic features that you may be able to identify include:

- **Speed of speech** – is the pace fast or slow?
- **Tone of voice** – high- or low-pitched?
- **Flow** – is the speech flowing or stilted?
- **Volume** – is the speaker quiet or loud?
- **Intonation** – is their speech animated or flat?
- **Clarity** – are the words clear or mumbled?
- **Fitted pauses** – are they using 'ums', 'ers', grunts and gasps?
- **Silence** – is there a torrent of words or are there long gaps?

A negative tone can have detrimental effects, for example, an angry voice is less likely to be successful in persuading a patient to undergo treatment. Conversely, a positive voice, with a warm, friendly tone, enables patients to ask questions, engage in discussion, trust their diagnosis and follow instructions about treatment. Nishizawa *et al.* (2006) found that in interactions with a simulated patient, student nurses used less non-verbal cues than trained nurses. For example, 90 per cent remained standing so could not readily meet the patient's gaze and they used less hand gesturing. This suggests that nurses need training to improve their own use of non-verbal communication (NVC) and their facilitation of NVC in others.

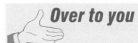

Over to you

Earlier we talked about ambiguity in spoken language. Working in pairs, repeat these phrases in different ways, changing the tone or emphasis. What different interpretations does this lead to?

- You can do that.
- Why won't you take these?
- How did you end up like that?
- We will come and do it later.

Finally, consider how many of the words below would describe the kinds of expression that you used:

- Pleading
- Instructional
- Encouraging
- Annoyed
- Questioning
- Confident
- Positive

Facial expression

Our faces are very expressive. Beyond obvious cues to emotions such as tears, the facial muscles enable us to move our mouths, eyes, eyebrows and fore-heads, both voluntarily and involuntarily, indicating to others how we feel. Matsumoto and Ekman (1989) found that the production and interpretation of the most common facial expressions is very similar across different cul-tural backgrounds: anywhere in the world, smiling means that a person is happy. These expressions seem to be spontaneous rather than acquired. People who have been blind from birth, so cannot have learned by copying others, display the same facial expressions for these basic emotions as sighted people (Galati *et al.* 1997).

Our facial expressions are important for others to understand us. When they are absent, such as in telephone calls, judging emotional state is more difficult.

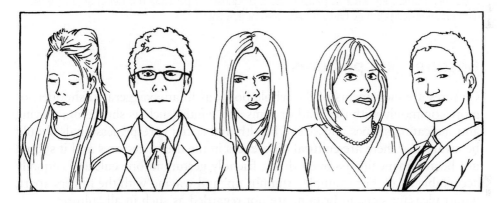

Can you understand how these people are feeling from their faces?

Gaze

Eye contact tells us a listener is paying attention and can indicate expectation, concern or sincerity. Prolonged eye contact, however, is threatening.

Gaze also helps with turn-taking in conversation. We tend to look directly at the other person when we have finished speaking, indicating that they may begin. If we pause, intending to continue, we tend to look down. Eye contact thus says we are about to stop (or start) speaking. When this regulation breaks down – for example over the telephone or if somebody persistently interrupts – communication is less effective.

Unlike facial expressions, the role of eye contact in communication is culturally dependent. The use of eye contact to regulate turn-taking is typical of British and American spoken language. By convention, in some cultures women do not make eye contact with men except in intimate situations; in others, social status dictates whether eye contact is appropriate.

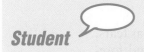

Student

Second year student physiotherapist

Talking about talking

Q: When you talk to patients, do you think it is important that they can see your face?
A: I think it's really important.

Q: Why?
A: Because I always think you can tell a lot from facial expressions, like whether patients are in pain. It's also polite to look people in the face.

Q: What do you do to try to ensure that they can see you easily?
A: Sometimes I crouch down to the person's level, if they are sat in a chair.

Q: Do you think that you ever have to try to mask your facial expressions and if so why might this be important?
A: I have had to do this. Particularly when a patient has a diagnosis of possibly not being able to walk unaided again that I know about but they haven't been told of this yet.

Gestures and postures

Gestures are movements of the whole body, as in an exaggerated shudder, or more commonly with the head or arms and hands (such as shrugging, waving and indicating shapes and sizes). Health and social care professionals should be aware that there are cultural differences in the use of gestures and it should not be automatically assumed that a friendly gesture in one culture is equally acceptable to all. For example, 'thumbs up' and waving with the fingers apart, whilst pleasant signs in Britain, are not regarded as such in all cultures.

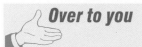

Over to you

The next time you have a day-to-day conversation with a friend or member of your family, try standing back to back with them and let your arms lie by your sides. See how long you can keep going before you try to express yourself using your hands!

Postures are static body positions. Sitting (or standing) up straight or, alternatively, slouching, are two postures that convey opposite messages. A formal, upright posture is assertive, a slumped position more passive. An 'open' posture is one in which the limbs are held relatively far from the body, arms hanging to the sides or stretched out on a table. In a 'closed' posture the limbs are held in, as if to 'protect' the body, for example with the arms folded or legs crossed beneath the body. Open postures indicate confidence; closed ones insecurity. Leaning forwards, towards another person, may indicate confidence or friendliness but can also appear to be aggressive.

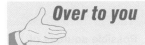

Over to you

Record a TV discussion programme and watch it with the sound turned down. Use a pre-written sheet with 30-second intervals marked down the margin. Try to record examples of non-verbal communication. Try to identify the emotions being expressed and note them alongside the time. Watch the video again, this time with the sound on. Did you correctly interpret the emotions from the non-verbal information alone?

Touch and personal space

We have, around our bodies, an invisible 'bubble', our **personal space**, into which we accept invasion from particular individuals. The more intimate our relationship with the person, the further they may enter into our personal space. Hall (1966) identified four zones based on the distances individuals tolerate with different relationships (Table 2.3). The ranges of these zones vary with social factors such as culture, gender and age, with some groups being more tolerant of people standing close to them and of gestures involving touch. Gleeson and Higgins (2009) investigated the use of touch by psychiatric nurses and found that physical touch needed to be sensitive to the patient's needs and to respect their personal space and cultural background. For example, males raised concerns that touching females could be misinterpreted as a sexual advance. As a consequence, they were more cautious and minimal in their use of touch, doing so only in a public space, where others could see the interaction.

In a hospital setting, maintaining personal space for patients may be difficult. Conversations that patients may feel should be confined to an intimate zone may be audible to others on a ward – even when curtains are drawn around the bed. Ideally, such conversations would be conducted in a separate room but this may not be practical on a busy ward or safe with patients whose mobility is limited. In order to provide such patients with a sense of privacy, curtains may be drawn, but this is illusory – they are not soundproof. It is worth observing that, for some patients, their own bed is perceived as a 'safe place' and they would prefer to remain there.

When communicating with patients in a confined space, nurses should maintain a distance at which they can be easily heard without being intimidating. Remember how invasive you find people standing close to you in a queue. Sitting at the same height as the patient helps to avoid the sensation of crowding them and sitting at an angle is less confrontational than positioning yourself directly face-to-face.

Touch is a very intimate non-verbal signal often used to indicate affection, for example through hugging, stroking and tickling. For individuals outside intimate relationships, bodily contact is limited and when it exists, such as in shaking hands, it is highly ritualized. This formality allows a degree of bodily contact that would otherwise be uncomfortable with a

Personal space
The area an individual maintains between themselves and others, which varies according to factors such as the intimacy of the relationship, circumstance and culture

Table 2.3 Personal space zones			
Zone	**Distance (metres)**	**Typical relationships and behaviours**	**Possible sources of communication**
Intimate	0–0.5 x 4 m	Contact is intimate (e.g. between sexual partners, comforting someone with a hug or treating a patient)	Touch is the predominant means of communication, although smell and skin temperature may be informative
Personal	0.5–1.2 m	Contact is close (e.g. between friends, encounters in shops, talking to a patient in bed, chair or a ward)	Speech is the main communication channel, accompanied by paralinguistic and non-verbal cues. Touch can still be used
Social	1.2–3.7 m	People maintain a distance from each other (e.g. in business situations, small meetings, spoken consultations in an office or across a desk)	Speech is the main communication channel, touch is no longer available but other non-verbal cues can be used
Public	13.7 m	Formal settings such as giving a presentation or speaking at a large meeting	Speech, sometimes amplified, is the main communication channel. The greater the distance the less the recipient can gain from non-verbal cues

stranger. However, nurses need to fulfil a supportive role and this is often enhanced by the use of subtle physical contact. This must be well judged to avoid being invasive but can effectively indicate attention and offer encouragement, or reassurance. A balance is needed between the two. In the process of caring for patients' health there is necessarily a need for bodily contact and nurses should remain aware that, for each new patient, this has the potential to cause unease.

Appearance

Clothing, hairstyle and presentation are aspects of our appearance. Many roles and settings within the health and social care profession have dress codes or policies relating to standards of appearance. The way a nurse appears can convey several messages.

Most obviously, a uniform indicates role. This is helpful for patients at a practical level as they then know who is who. However, a uniform can also play an important role in reassuring patients, who are in a strange environment surrounded by people they may never have met. An individual who is not confident about having a blood sample taken in his local surgery may be reassured by the nurse's uniform. For example, Brosky *et al.* (2003) found that the clothing worn by dental care providers affected the comfort and anxiety experienced by their patients. Conversely, casual clothes may send messages about a lack of care, cleanliness or respect. However, consider what benefits there might be, if staff on children's wards wear less formal clothing. An investigation of patients' preferences for different nurses' uniforms, found that this depended on age (Albert *et al.* 2008). Older adult patients felt nurses in white uniforms were more professional (than those with a small print, bold print or solid colour) but paediatric patients and younger adults had no significant uniform preference. Health and social care staff must also be aware that they should not stereotype patients on the basis of their appearance.

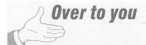

Over to you

A health and social care student was denied a placement because she had three tongue piercings. She challenged the decision on the basis that she had clear plastic retainer studs that were acceptable to her other employer, a supermarket, where she worked on the delicatessen. She was told that they were unhygienic, to which she replied with her letter from her dentist indicating her high level of oral health.

Do you think these steps were appropriate? Imagine the perspective of an elderly patient, a young patient themselves or a patient with mouth cancer. What decision would you have made?

KEY POINTS

- When we speak to someone, there are three parts to the message, the linguistic (meaning of the words), paralinguistic (pitch and volume of voice, pace of, etc.) and non-verbal communication (e.g. postures and gestures). In addition to the message conveyed by the words, the other elements are useful indicators of emotional state or attitude.

- When you have to invade a patient's personal space try to strike a balance between formality to help allow the patient to recognize that the procedure is a necessary part of their care and informality to offer reassurance.

- A smart appearance, especially your uniform, reassures many patients, although for a minority it may be intimidating.

- To avoid drawing conclusions based on your first impressions of patients, this is discriminatory and will not ensure fair treatment.

FACTORS AFFECTING COMMUNICATION

A wide range of factors affects communication, including:

- emotional state – of all communicators, not just the patient
- social and cultural factors – such as stereotypes, language barriers and social class
- age – differences in communication and expectations of the young and older adults
- gender – male and female patients, as well as nurses, differ in communication style
- confidentiality – the effects of trust and privacy.

Emotions

We have seen that we can judge a patient's emotion from their facial expressions to help us in interacting. Some emotions, however, can act as barriers to communication.

Reflective activity

Write a list of health issues that could make patients feel:

- Angry
- Fearful
- Shocked
- Anxious
- Embarrassed
- Guilty
- Isolated
- Confused

Think of different situations in which you have felt each of the above emotions strongly. Write an account of any problems you experienced when trying to communicate with others on these occasions.

Consider how patients could suffer the effects you may have experienced in other contexts.

The emotions of health and social care professionals are also important. Jeffery (1979) observed that staff might hold negative attitudes towards patients with problems considered to be medically 'trivial', especially when the patients are drunk, homeless or appear to have taken a drug overdose as an attention-seeking behaviour. Such opinions would reduce empathy with the patient. Nurses' attitudes are sometimes more positive than doctors'. Ramon *et al.*

(1975) found that when working with cases of self-poisoning, although doctors were sympathetic towards those they considered to have 'depressive' suicidal motives, they were less so to those patients they perceived to have 'manipulative' motives. Nurses, in contrast, were more accepting and sympathetic. Indeed, when patients view their symptoms as trivial (even though they might not be), nurses can provide a more effective service than doctors, for example with elderly patients who do not want to 'bother' the doctor with problems such as constipation, headaches and rashes (Lucker *et al.*, 1998). The role of the emotional component in prejudice is explored further later on.

Social and cultural factors

In the last section we considered some cultural similarities and differences in communication that could relate to many different kinds of interaction. There are also health-related cultural differences, for instance whether an individual perceives symptoms as important, their choice of treatment and whether they seek professional health and social care at all. When it is culturally unacceptable to complain about pain at home, this may affect the likelihood of expressing this, and other concerns about symptoms or future health, to staff in hospital.

Practitioners may make mistakes in interactions because they make stereotyped assumptions about their patients or lack cultural knowledge. For example, El-Amouri and O'Neill (2011) proposed 'culturally competent care' and gave examples of patients being misunderstood. A Haitian patient with abdominal pain was admitted to a mental health ward by mistake as she was performing cultural rituals that involved speaking loudly to spirits. In another case, an Arab patient believed her breast milk was unfit for her baby and wanted the nurse to check it, whilst the nurse wanted her to feed the baby.

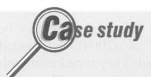

Case study

Stereotyped assumptions

A female patient, with long-term dysmenorrhoea, who was on holiday away from her normal surgery was in such pain that she was taken to the local doctor. The GP was helpful and friendly, and was appropriately determining possible causes of the pain, but was misled by stereotypical thinking. Part of the dialogue went as follows:

GP: Could you be pregnant?
Patient: No.

GP: Are you sexually active?
Patient: Yes.
GP: What method of contraception are you using?
Patient: None.
GP: So you could be pregnant then?
Patient: No.
GP: But you are sexually active?
Patient: Yes.
GP: And you haven't been sterilized?
Patient: (who, by this time, is on the verge of passing out) No.
GP: So you could be pregnant then?
Patient: No I couldn't – she's my partner (indicating the person who had brought her to the surgery).

An additional issue to consider in assessing the adequacy of health and social care provision is whether communication is being conducted in the patient's, or the professional's, first language. Many health services provide printed information in several languages (e.g. in Wales, leaflets are available in English and in Welsh). For face-to-face consultations, however, interpreters may be required if the patient's symptoms are to be correctly understood and they are to receive adequate information about their diagnosis and choice about their care. This is important for both patients and staff. Leininger (2002) notes that confusion, disorientation and distress can be caused to nurses when patients don't respond to them in culturally familiar ways.

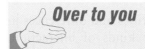

Over to you

Barriers to communication

You may have first-hand experience of trying to communicate in a second language, if not this is a useful exercise to help you to experience what it is like to be unable to find the words to express yourself. You will need to work with a partner. Write out the alphabet in large letters across the middle of a piece of paper. Fold the paper in half so that you can only see either the first or the last half of the alphabet. Using only words that begin with letters in the half of the alphabet you can see, trying to tell your partner about yourself, where you live, what you like doing, how you are going to spend your weekend. Swap roles between speaker and listener and use the other half of the alphabet.

How did you get on? Probably, you knew exactly what you wanted to say; it was 'in your head' but you couldn't find a way to explain it.

If you have not yet studied reflective practice, you might find Jasper M. *Beginning Reflective Practice* (2012) useful.

Finally, even for patients operating in their first language, there may be differences between sectors of society. Janssen *et al.* (2004) investigated whether the written complexity of materials mattered. They tested men with higher and lower levels of education with simplified information and targeted information (intended to help with specific problems, such as coping with difficult situations). Simplification made no difference, but with the lower educational attainers, targeted materials were more effective in producing behavioural change. This suggests making material relevant, as well as understandable, is important to changing health behaviour.

Evidence also suggests that patients from lower SES groups may be disadvantaged with regard to health and social care. For example, Wilson (2009) found that nurses were more likely to take notice of higher SES patients' views about their pain level and preferred pain management. In a study of rehabilitation following hip fractures, Freburger *et al.* (2012) found that individuals of lower SES received fewer hours of care per day than those of higher SES.

Age

People from different generations have grown up in different social worlds so effectively form separate subcultural groups. In this respect they may have differing beliefs, attitudes and knowledge in relation to health and health and social care. Of course, many patients will not conform to the stereotypical member of their age-related group and to assume so would be discriminatory. Nevertheless, differences have been identified in the relationships between health and social care professionals and patients of different ages. Some research suggests that there is a communication advantage for older patients, some that advancing age is a disadvantage.

As we get older our cognitive abilities change: our vocabulary and general communication skills improve, however, our memories tend to get worse. Older patients are poorer at recalling information about drug dosage (Kiernan and Issacs, 1981) and need shorter, more concise messages if they are to recall effectively (Forshaw, 2002). With older patients, the use of a patient-centred style of communication leads to greater satisfaction (Peck, 2011).

Effective communication with children may require different skills because they are less able to describe their thoughts and feelings, or do so differently from adults. Children also differ in their understanding of health and illness. Bibace and Walsh (1979) described the changing conception of health through childhood (Table 2.4). For example, children in the phenomenistic stage (0–3 years) may believe that being naughty caused them to be ill. This may be unintentionally reinforced if they are hospitalized and think they have been sent away from their family as a punishment.

Table 2.4 The changing understanding of health and illness through childhood			
Stage	**Age (years)**	**Description**	**Effect on communication**
Phenomenistic stage	0–3	The child associates illness with one specific (and often unrelated) 'cause' such as 'Grandma gave me tummy ache' because it happened to start at Grandma's house. They may also focus on one symptom, such as 'Asthma is coughing'	The child may therefore fail to report all the symptoms they are experiencing or ignore the actual cause (if this is unknown to the carers)
Contagion stage	3–7	The child grasps the idea that diseases can be transmitted from one person to another but may over-generalize both the kinds of condition that are infections e.g. 'Did you catch your broken arm from your brother?') and the methods of transmission (e.g. believing they can catch measles from a friend over the telephone)	The child fails to recognize an actual route of infection so will not report it

(Continued)

Table 2.4 The changing understanding of health and illness through childhood *(Continued)*			
Stage	**Age (years)**	**Description**	**Effect on communication**
Contamination stage	7 onwards	The child comprehends the causation of disease by agents such as germs and that these are conveyed by some medium (e.g. the air). They also recognize that diseases have a range of symptoms	The child's ability to report their bodily sensations and possible causative agents improves
Internalization stage	7–11	The child begins to grasp the relationship between health (or illness) and behaviour, and that the consequences affect the body on the inside. For example they may describe the effects of cigarette smoke as 'bad for your lungs' or say that eating too many sweets can rot your teeth	The child is more likely to be able to follow health advice as the impact of their own actions on their own health is understood
Physiological stage	11 onwards	Factors such as the child's exposure to education increases understanding about body structure, e.g. organs, and both its function and dysfunction. This enables the child to see that there may be many factors that affect health	The child will be increasingly capable of understanding scientific explanations of the cause and effects of their own illnesses or those of others if these are given in terms they are familiar with. Prior to this, the child may be unable to understand the purpose of these treatments and when these are unpleasant, may become confused and upset
Psycho-physiological stage	12–14	In this final stage, the child begins to comprehend the role of both physical and physiological factors in health, e.g. that stress can make people physically ill and that being unwell can be a source of stress	Children at this stage will also be able to follow logical, reasoned arguments so will be better able to enter into discussions about alternative treatments

Even though an ill child's understanding may be limited they should still be given information about their illness and treatment as research shows that this is beneficial. For example, nurses should explain what procedures will feel like and how long they will last, and give children the opportunity to express their feelings and ask questions. Specific techniques can also reduce distress. In a review of randomized controlled trials, Chambers *et al.* (2009) identified breathing exercises, child-directed distraction, nurse-led distraction and cognitive-behavioural techniques as effective in reducing the pain and distress experienced by children receiving immunizations. Interestingly, Zuwala and Barber (2001) found that providing information for parents (a video demonstrating the use of an inhalation mask) was effective in helping to reduce child distress during preoperative anaesthesia.

The communication of honest information is also important for terminally ill children, who, like terminally ill adults, tend to have a better understanding of the seriousness of their condition than health and social care professionals believe. The death of a child is traumatic for the adults involved, both staff and parents, so the child often receives less information than an adult would. This exclusion can prevent the child from expressing their fears or asking questions, so they may harbour distressing (and incorrect) beliefs. Martinson (1995) observes that terminally ill children know they are dying. They are aware, perhaps even more acutely than adults, of their loss of movement, energy and enthusiasm. She identifies the importance of listening to the child and considering their needs, for example recognizing that children are often under-medicated despite experiencing the same degree of pain as adults.

Children whose parents are dying also need special attention with regard to communication. Adults often feel the need to protect children but failing to tell a child that a parent is dying does not avert fear, indeed it denies the child access to the information and emotional support they need. Longfield and Warnick (2009) observe that nurses are in a unique position to help children in this situation by communicating with them.

Gender

Research has found that often health and social care professionals see patients in gender stereotyped ways and that this affects their care. For example, in a simulation, McDonald and Bridge (1991) found that female patients would be given fewer painkillers and less time was anticipated for emotional support when planning for their care. Such differences are also found in studies of actual patient care. Foss and Sundby (2003) found that nurses describe female patients as more demanding than males, although unlike physicians, nurses perceived young women to be most demanding, rather than elderly ones. Such perceptions about women tending to exaggerate demands can also directly affect care. Calderone (1990) found that nurses controlling post-operative pain medication offered pain medication more frequently to male patients, and sedative medication more frequently to females. We will discuss gender stereotypes and prejudice further later on.

RESEARCH IN BRIEF

Chong (2012) Gender preference and implications for screening colonoscopy

Aim: To investigate patients' gender preferences for nursing staff during endoscopy and its impact on acceptance for screening colonoscopy (SC).

Procedure: Patients attending clinics were invited to participate. Questionnaires asked about whether they would go for a SC if they had appropriate indications (such as age over 50 years, family history of colorectal cancer, anaemia, rectal bleeding, loss of appetite, weight loss or abdominal pain); about their preferences for the gender of the endoscopists and assistants; and whether they would still attend SC if their preferences were not met.

Findings: From 470 completed questionnaires, more female than male participants expressed a gender preference (70 per cent compared to 62.8 per cent), with female patients strongly preferring female endoscopists and male patients predominantly preferring male endoscopists. The same pattern was seen for gender preference for nurses (see graph below). A third of participants said they would decline an SC if their gender preferences were not met – even if they had appropriate indications and this pattern was more evident for female patients.

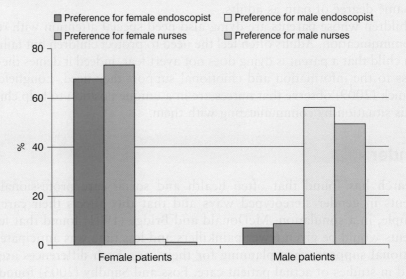

Conclusion: Gender preference for endoscopy nurses is more important than for endoscopists, especially for female patients, which has implications for the success of screening programmes.

Confidentiality

You will have considered the need for confidentiality and the rights of patients in the health and social care setting. Confidentiality also plays a role in communication as patients need to trust their nurses not to divulge their personal information to others.

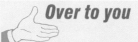

Over to you

Read the following examples and consider how the individuals' beliefs about confidentiality would affect communication with the patient or colleague.

- Ahmed has an appointment with his college nurse for a BCG booster. He is worried about it making him ill as he has recently taken some Ecstasy. He wants to tell the nurse but is scared his teachers will be told.
- Jagdeep is having a sexual relationship with her boyfriend and wants to go to her GP for the contraceptive pill. She is only 15.
- Eileen has terminal cancer and is dying. She tells her nurse that she doesn't want to talk to her family but she appears to be very lonely.
- Helen who is 7 months pregnant has just discovered that her partner is having an affair and is really embarrassed and depressed about it. She has asked the midwife not to tell anyone.
- Greg and Alice have both started working as newly qualified social workers. Greg is upset about the living conditions of one of his patient's families, and disagrees with his supervisor's statement that it is not really that bad, compared to others. Greg moans to Alice, but has asked her not to say anything in case his supervisor and fellow social workers think he is interfering.

To protect individuals from vulnerability, four categories of information need to be kept confidential:

1 **identity** – e.g. name, address, marital status
2 **medical history** – e.g. the nature and progression of diseases and treatments
3 **social circumstances** – e.g. family, sexual orientation, housing, employment
4 **psychological factors** – e.g. details of emotional state, stress levels and mental health.

Any placement or employer should make you aware of their code of conduct with regard to ethical issues such as confidentiality. From the perspective of the service user, confidentiality is important because it provides a level of security without which patients (and staff too) may feel insufficiently confident to express themselves fully. The information with which health and social care professionals are trusted should therefore be treated with respect. Individuals may fear the process and consequences of disclosure; they may feel that they will be judged or discriminated against on the basis of information they have divulged or that, if misused, even simple facts such as their being in hospital could put them at risk from, for instance, burglary.

Reflective activity

Good communication

Think of an instance when you have engaged in or observed in interaction between a patient and a health and social care professional that demonstrated good communication skills. Briefly describe the scene and comment on what communication skills, such as choice of words, non-verbal cues and appearance helped the communicator to transmit their message effectively. Think about the ways in which the health and social care professional facilitated communication to the patient: Was there an attempt to put the patient at ease? Did they ask questions? If so were they open or closed? Did they interrupt the patient?

Special needs in communication

The most important thing you need to remember about communicating with people with special communication needs is that all the same rules apply! You will need to make sure that you are aware of the communication cycle:

- Is your message clear enough?
- Is your message being received?
- Are you receiving feedback?

If the answer to any of these questions is 'no', then you need a course of action to remedy the situation, bearing in mind that the later stages of the cycle cannot happen without the earlier ones. You will need to consider what you can do, or what resources (human or artificial) might make the message more effective – the answer may be very simple, such as gaining the attention of a deaf person who can lip-read before you start to speak. Finally, ask yourself whether there really is no feedback – you may be able to detect a gesture, or a change in expression or in posture that is indicating a reply. You can then build on this to verify the individual's response.

The obvious special needs that affect communication, such as sensory impairments, are not the only possibilities. People with learning difficulties such as Down's syndrome or autism may find communication difficult, as may people with acquired problems such brain injury or Parkinson's disease. The requirements for communicating with people with learning difficulties will vary for different individuals. However, always try to:

- Speak directly to the person themselves, not their carer.
- Express yourself in a clear, simple way without being patronizing.
- Be prepared to repeat questions and to wait for and listen carefully to the answer.

Some impairments to communication can be assisted with human or technological aids. One that you should be aware of is deafness. Many people with hearing impairments can communicate effectively given appropriate opportunities and/or resources. For example, a deaf person who is fluent in sign language does not have a problem with understanding or being the sender or receiver in a communication cycle – provided that they have access to a sign interpreter. People with hearing impairments use a range of strategies to assist their communication. Look at Table 2.5 to see how you can help.

Speaking to a person with a visual impairment should be no different from speaking to a sighted person; speaking loudly or slowly is unnecessary and inappropriate. However, it is important to ensure that you have been recognized, so introduce yourself and anyone else who is with you. Also, try to be aware of the missing aspects of communication for a person with a visual impairment and inform them verbally, for example, if you are leaving the room for a while, and intend to make physical contact, which might be a shock.

Autistic spectrum disorders
A range of pervasive developmental problems characterized by difficulties with social interaction and communication and a tendency for the individual to show restricted and repetitive behaviour patterns

Table 2.5 Communication strategies for people with hearing loss	
Communication strategy	**What can I do?**
Lip-reading	Ensure that you are facing the person, that your face is in good light and that it is not obscured (e.g. by your hands). Don't exaggerate your speech; be prepared to repeat yourself or rephrase your statements
British sign language	Locate a sign interpreter if one is available. Direct your questions and answers to the person themselves, not the interpreter
Fingerspelling	Use fingerspelling if necessary but remember that it relies on being able to spell and deaf people may not necessarily be very familiar with written English if their education has been delayed
Hearing aids	Be aware that a hearing aid may not provide full hearing: a user may be employing other strategies, such as lip reading, and may find hearing when there is background noise, such as on a busy ward, more difficult than in a quiet environment. Do not shout, because this distorts your voice and makes lip-reading more difficult

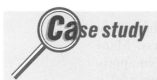

Case study

Working with a patient with an Autistic Spectrum Disorder (ASD)

A young man with an Autistic Spectrum Disorder (ASD) visits the Accident and Emergency Department with his carer having tripped and fallen injuring his wrist. His verbal communication skills are limited. During nurse assessment they are told that his injury is a low priority and he will need to wait a considerable time to see a doctor. The waiting area is very crowded and the room is noisy. He sits down for a few minutes then begins to pace up and down. After 20 minutes he becomes extremely agitated and distressed. A member of staff approaches the patient looking rather cross and tells him that if he continues to cause disruption he will have to leave the department. She rather sternly asks if he wants to leave to which he replies 'yes'.

1 What factors might alert a health professional to the fact that the patient has an ASD and/or learning disability?

2 What are the barriers to effective communication for this patient?

3 What stereotypical assumptions might health professionals make about a young man who appears agitated?

4 How might the health professional have improve her communication with the young man?

Note: Children and adults with autism lack the ability to understand the mental states of others so find it difficult to understand other people's emotions and to interpret their behaviour. This is one reason that they have difficulty with social situations, as in the absence of understanding the emotions of others, their behaviour is less predictable.

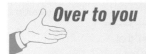

Over to you

A confident lip-reader can follow a great deal of what is being said if the speaker's face is in good light, if they are not exaggerating their speech and if the words are familiar. However, some sounds cannot be differentiated from the lips alone, so context has to be used to 'fill the gaps'. This exercise demonstrates the difficulties.

Working with a partner, say list A using 'silent speech' (forming the words without using your voice). Swap roles and use list B.

List A	List B
1 Slow	11 Sheet
2 Go	12 Cheat
3 Jeer	13 Lip
4 Sheer	14 Rip
5 Chew	15 Chum
6 Goo	16 Come
7 Bright	17 Clues
8 Blight	18 Choose
9 Cheap	19 Jaw
10 Jeans	20 Sure

KEY POINTS

- The patient's emotions, and your own, are important in effective communication. Be aware patients are ill and possibly nervous so will find interaction more difficult.
- Social, cultural and gender stereotypes can lead to bias in care, which is inappropriate.
- Patients of different age may differ in their expectations of communication and need for interaction.
- Patients have a right to confidentiality and this is important to give them confidence to communicate effectively.
- When dealing with patients with special needs, pay particular attention to whether your communications have been received and understood.

EVALUATING INTERACTIONS

Evaluating the psychological aspects of a situation is a key way to improve the effectiveness of your own interactions. If you have used *Beginning Reflective Practice* (Jasper, 2012) in this series, you will be familiar with reflecting on your own experiences.

Some questions to ask yourself when evaluating communication skills include:

- Was the interaction patient-centred or professional-centred?
- What role was played by different communication skills?

  - Verbal aspects of speech:
      Questions – were open/closed questions used effectively?
  - Level/jargon – did the content inform or exclude the patient?
  - Non-verbal aspects of speech: volume, tone, pace – were these used appropriately?
  - Listening skills: active listening, use of mirroring, empathy and silence – were these used sufficiently and sensitively?
  - Other non-verbal communication: facial expressions, eye contact, gestures, postures, touch, appearance – were these appropriate to the context in choice and extent?
  - Physical aspects such as seating, privacy – did the receiver feel secure?

- Were there any barriers to communication?

  - What were they? Consider:

    Leading questions
    Effects of emotions such as fear or embarrassment
    Impairments and special needs
    Invasion of personal space

Gender
Age
Social factors
Cultural factors
Time available
Language or dialect

- – Were any barriers recognized by (all of) the communicators?
- – Was an attempt made to overcome them?
- – How was this attempted?
- – Was the attempt successful?

● If a similar situation arose again, would you act differently?

- – What would you do differently?
- – Why?

The main reason for evaluating communication is in order to improve it, so it is important that, through the reflective process, you recognize what you have gained or learned from different situations.

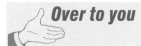

Over to you

You can explore the influence of effective and ineffective communication through role-play. Try the following situations:

● A physiotherapist with a patient who has been undergoing the same treatment for a long time.

● A health visitor embarking on their first session with a new patient.

● A plaster technician, who is trying to gain the co-operation of a patient who is finding the procedure painful.

● A student radiographer being mentored by a very experienced radiographer.

CONCLUSIONS

Successful health and social care, at any level, relies on effective communication between professionals and patients and between health and social care staff. In this chapter we have considered a range of factors that affect communication. Some, such as the practitioner–patient relationship and the use of medical jargon, are specific to health and social care settings and many others, such as non-verbal communication and personal space, can arise in any encounter. For nurses, attention to communication is particularly important as patients may, for a variety of reasons, be unable to communicate effectively, yet the need for their understanding and response may be crucial for their well-being. In addition, communication plays an important supporting role in recovery.

By exploring the issues raised by different factors in interactions we have considered ways to improve communication where barriers exist. In addition, we have looked at specific ways to enhance communication in instances where barriers are permanent and specific, such as for patients with sensory impairments or learning difficulties.

Reflective activity

Try to recall the details of two difficult but contrasting interactions between patients and health and social care professionals in which you engaged or that you observed. Choose one that you feel was an example of effectively used communication skills in which barriers were overcome and another that was less successful because communication problems were not resolved. Picture the scenes and consider how the sender and receiver might have felt in each and how, in turn, these feelings would have impacted on the communication itself. If a less experienced student than yourself were going to find himself/herself faced with a similar situation in the future, what advice would you give them?

RAPID RECAP

Check your progress so far by working through each of the following questions.

1 What is the communication cycle?

2 What is meant by 'patient-centred' and 'practitioner-centred' approaches to interaction?

3 What does the acronym SURETY stand for?

If you have difficulty with any of the questions, read through the section again to refresh your understanding before moving on.

KEY REFERENCES

Other references are listed on the supporting website.

Brady, M. (2009) Hospitalized children's view of the good nurse. *Nurse Ethics* 16 (5): 545–560.

Chong, V.H. (2012) Gender preference and implications for screening colonoscopy: impact of endoscopy nurses. *World Journal of Gastroenterology* 18 (27): 3590–3594.

Department of Health (2010) Essence of Care 2010, *Benchmarks for the Fundamental Aspects of Care*, TSO (The Stationery Office), London.

Jasper, M. *Beginning Reflective Practice* (2012), Nursing and Healthcare Practice Series, Cengage EMEA, Andover.

CHAPTER 3

PSYCHOLOGY AND THE INDIVIDUAL IN HEALTH AND SOCIAL CARE SETTINGS

PERSONALITY

What personality traits affect people in health and social care settings?

The type A personality

Two doctors, Friedman and Rosenman, began their research into personality with a casual observation of the state of their waiting room furniture. The pattern of wear on the chairs was unusual; rather than wearing on the seat, the front edge and arms had worn out first. They later observed that their coronary patients tended to sit on the edge of their seat, leaping up frequently to enquire how much longer they would be kept waiting for their appointments. The possibility of a connection between the heart conditions and the tense, frenetic behaviour of these individuals led to the proposal of 'hurry sickness', later renamed 'type A behaviour' (Friedman and Rosenman, 1974).

It is possible to classify people into personality types on the basis of patterns of behaviour. Type A individuals tend to be highly competitive, aggressive, impatient and hostile, with a strong urge for success. Their behaviour tends to be goal directed and performed at speed. In contrast, people with type B behaviour are relatively laid back, lacking the urgency and drive typical of type A individuals. Some individuals do not fall clearly into either category and are termed type X.

The risk of stress-related illnesses, such as coronary heart disease, is greater for type A individuals than for type B (Rosenman *et al.*, 1975, Haynes *et al.*, 1980). Type A behaviour of itself may not necessarily cause stress; individuals with this personality type may tend to expose themselves to more stressful situations, such as high-pressure jobs, or may experience situations such as queuing as more annoying. Even if the cause is psychological, the effect must be still be mediated by a biological process. One significant difference in this respect is hostility. The tendency for people displaying type A behaviours to be aggressive may lead them to experience more conflicts with others, for example when driving. Several studies (e.g. Perry and Baldwin, 2000) have found that type A behaviours are associated with aggression on the road.

A possible physiological route of action is the **neurohormonal** system, specifically the effects of hormone levels on **atherosclerosis**. Type A individuals show elevated heart rate, blood pressure, skin conductance and catecholamine response. These are all changes associated with stress, resembling chronic activation of the sympathetic adrenal medullary system.

Not all studies demonstrate a clear relationship between stress and type A behaviour. Freeman *et al.* (2000) predicted that the political violence in Northern Ireland would increase the stress experienced by members of the population and it would be expected that individuals demonstrating type A behaviours would be more severely affected. However, when Freeman *et al.* compared stress levels in groups of dental students from Belfast in 1992 and during the 1994–96 ceasefire, they found no effect related to type A behaviour. The students' personality did not seem to affect their experience of stress, although other factors, such as gender and social support, were important.

Hardiness

Kobasa (1979) studied the stress levels, personalities and health of executives. She found that, of those who were highly stressed, the individuals who did or did not become ill differed in terms of a personality factor she called **hardiness**. There are three key characteristics of a hardy personality. These are:

Neurohormonal Events or sequences involving interaction between the nervous and endocrine systems

Atherosclerosis Hardening of the arteries due to fatty deposits lining the inside walls of the vessels

Hardiness A trait used to describe people who appear to be able to withstand emotional and psychological stress even in the long term)

- **Commitment** – a sense of purpose and involvement in events and activities.
- **Control** – a belief that one can influence events in one's own life.
- **Challenge** – a perception of change as positive and representing an opportunity for growth rather than a threat.

The hardy executives were less ill, perhaps because they treated problems as potentially beneficial and therefore less stressful. As a result they may take more direct action in the face of stress, such as problem-focused coping strategies, enabling them to tackle rather than avoid issues. Recent evidence suggests that a hardy personality may also reduce the likelihood of 'burnout' when under pressure (Sciacchitano *et al.*, 2001).

Korbasa's original study only looked at males, although subsequent investigations have demonstrated similar effects in women. Rhodewalt and Zone (1989) assessed the illness and depression ratings of women with high and low hardiness scores. They found that hardy women suffered lower rates of illness and depression following undesirable life changes than non-hardy women. The women also differed in their interpretation of life changes. High and low hardiness scorers experienced similar numbers of stressful events but more were classified as undesirable by the non-hardy group. This suggests that hardy individuals appraise potentially stressful events differently, buffering them against the negative effects of stress.

Hardiness may, however, be explained without recourse to special features of hardy people. First, it may be nothing more than positive **affect**. The effects of better coping might simply be explained by more positive appraisal and interpretation of events in the individual's life. Alternatively, hardiness may have an indirect rather than a direct effect on illness. 'Hardy' individuals may be more likely to engage in successful health-related behaviours, thus having a lower risk of illness.

Affect
In the context of psychology this refers to emotions or feelings

Locus of control

The way individuals appraise their role in controlling their own lives also appears to be important. Rotter (1966) identified a personality variable he called the **locus of control**. People who attribute control to factors they cannot govern, such as chance or the behaviour of other people, are described as having an external locus of control. Those who believe that they are responsible for themselves have an internal locus of control. This internal–external dimension may also relate to health behaviour. Strickland (1978) suggested that individuals with an internal locus of control may engage in more preventative measures, such as avoiding accidents and being informed about their own health.

The precise role of locus of control in the context of health has been investigated using the health locus of control (HLC) scale developed by Wallston *et al.* (1978). This measure, which looks specifically at an individual's beliefs about the factors that determine their health outcomes, assesses three dimensions:

Locus of control
The belief that someone has about how much control they or the environment have over their actions and behaviours)

- **Internal health locus of control** – the extent to which the individuals feel able to be responsible for their own health, for instance believing that 'the main thing that affects my health is what I myself do'.

- **Powerful others' control over health** – the individuals' belief in the role that other, important, people (such as doctors, nurses, family and friends) play in their health and holds views such as 'Whenever I don't feel well, I should consult a trained professional'.

- **Chance health locus of control** – the role that the individual assigns to pure 'luck' (or otherwise) and indicated by beliefs such as 'No matter what I do, if I am going to get sick, I will get sick'.

RESEARCH IN BRIEF

Steptoe and Wardle (2001) Locus of control and health behaviour

Aim: To investigate the relationship between health locus of control (HLC), health values and health-related behaviours in a diverse sample.

Procedure: A total of 4358 female and 2757 male university students aged 18–30 years from 18 European countries were tested on three measures: HLC, health values and ten health-related behaviours (physical exercise, not smoking, limited alcohol consumption, regular breakfast, daily tooth-brushing, seat-belt use and consumption of fruit, fat, fibre and salt).

Findings: There was a significant difference in the behaviours exhibited by individuals with the highest compared to the lowest internal HLC scores. Those with the lowest scores were 40 per cent more likely to engage in five of the health-compromising behaviours (exercise, daily tooth-brushing, eating fibre and avoiding salt and fat). Similarly, those with the highest chance HLC scores were 20 per cent less likely to select the healthy option for more than half of the behaviours (not smoking, limited alcohol consumption, regular breakfast, daily fruit, eating fibre and avoiding fat).

Conclusion: Low internal HLC and high chance HLC are associated with poor health choices. A low internal score suggests that the individual does not believe that they can affect their own health for the better, so they do not try. A high chance score indicates that the individual believes that factors outside their control influence their health and that their own efforts are therefore irrelevant.

Support for the HLC was also obtained by O'Carroll *et al.* (2001) in relation to the response of individuals who had suffered a myocardial infarction (heart attack). Many patients fail to request help when they are having a heart attack and O'Carroll *et al.* found that a high chance HLC was the best predictor of delay in seeking medical attention. Because these individuals believe that chance is a major factor determining their health they do not seek help soon enough and their delay, in these circumstances, could be fatal.

O'Carroll *et al.* suggest that attempts to modify the beliefs of people at risk could reduce their response time and therefore increase survival rates.

Many people engage in health-compromising behaviours, such as drug-taking, unprotected sex or overeating. Individuals with a high score on the chance dimension of HLC, whose beliefs suggest that whatever they do will have little effect on their health, would be expected to ignore risks to health. Hodgson (2001) used a student population to investigate perceived risk, risk-taking behaviour and HLC. The results showed a link between these variables, suggesting that for adolescents those who believe that their health status is determined by chance factors are more likely to engage in risky activities. This identifies a high risk group in terms of their age, occupation and beliefs and provides the basis for specifically targeted health education.

EMOTIONAL INTELLIGENCE

What is it?

Emotional intelligence
A person's ability to monitor their own emotions and the emotions of others correctly

Emotional Intelligence (EI) is basically a person's ability to monitor their own emotions and the emotions of others correctly. Then, we use this ability to guide our own thinking and behaviour. It appears to be focused around four ideas according to Salovey and Mayer (1990):

1. Perception of emotions – we need to do this correctly for both verbal and non-verbal emotional behaviour.
2. Reasoning based on these perceptions – we use the emotions to help us think about our own and others' behaviours and intentions.
3. Understanding these emotions – we need to fully understand why someone is acting, for example aggressively, before we react.
4. Managing these emotions – we need to be able to do this correctly and respond appropriately to people in social situations.

Over to you

Think about the following situation. You arrive at work on time but your boss is angry. Think of at least four possible reasons why they could be angry towards you?

How does it affect people who work in health and social care settings?

Kendall-Rayner (2012) noted that one university in Scotland was going to screen nursing applicants for EI. Part of this included assessing the emotions of a variety of faces giving reasons for their choices. Therefore, EI is now potentially becoming a priority in health and social care settings.

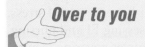

Over to you

Try this with a fellow health and social care trainee. Show different emotions through your face to see if the other person can correctly identify it. How easy/difficult was it?

There has been quite a lot of research looking at the role of EI in health and social care settings recently both in terms of health and social care professionals and health and social care professionals' leadership. Look back at the definition of EI and think about why it might be so important in health and social care settings before reading on.

RESEARCH IN BRIEF

van Dusseldorp *et al.* (2010) Emotional intelligence in mental health nurses.

Aim: To examine the level of EI in a sample of Dutch mental health nurses.

Method: The EI of a sample of 98 mental health nurses was measured using a self-report questionnaire called the Bar-On Emotional Quotient Inventory. They wanted to test out a variety of hypotheses, which included seeing if mental health nurses have higher than usual EI, testing if there were any gender differences in EI levels, whether the workplace affected EI levels and finally if EI was affected by age and experience.

Results: The mental health nurses did, on average, have a higher EI than the general Dutch population. There were no significant gender differences in EI overall but because EI was measured using different sub-scales, the research team could examine differences in these. Females scored higher on Interpersonal EI and Emotional Self-Awareness. There were also no differences in EI between those who worked in out-patient or inpatient facilities and EI was not correlated with age or level of experience.

Conclusion: A high level of EI is helpful for mental health nurses to be successful and cope with daily emotional demands in this particular health and social care setting. Interestingly, both males and females in this study could control emotional behaviours like frustration and aggression probably because they had elevated levels of EI. Finally, female nurses in this study tended to be better at 'establishing and maintaining satisfying professional relationships' (p. 560) than males.

EI has been linked to a variety of outcome measures in different studies. Beauvais *et al.* (2011) reported that in their sample of 87 nursing students in

America, EI was correlated with nursing performance – the higher the EI the better the student appeared to perform as a nurse. In addition, Por *et al.* (2011) discovered that in their sample of 130 nursing diploma students in the UK, EI was correlated with their general well-being, perceived competency as a nurse, problem-focused stress management and with lower levels of stress.

Codier *et al.* (2010) took a different approach to assessing EI and nursing. They examined 75 stories from a book published for nurses covering inspirational stories in nursing (Heacock, 2008). They scored each story on a number of dimensions, including if EI was present in them and whether EI linked to professionalism and performance as a nurse. Four researchers scored each story independently and for a concept to be recorded as being 'present', three of them had to have logged it. The main findings were:

- All but two stories had reference to EI somewhere in it (280 counts of EI were recorded in the 73 stories).
- Empathy, problem-solving and emotional self-awareness were the top three EI components mentioned in the stories. We focus on empathy later in this chapter.
- Scores of professionalism were correlated positively with EI content scores, so those that showed more EI were rated as being more professional.

Therefore, even in literature about nursing there is a focus on EI and its positive attributes on nursing professionalism.

One study did examine EI in just male nurses (Serap and Rahsan, 2011). A total of 87 male nurses in Turkey completed questionnaires measuring EI and also Leadership and whilst EI was only moderate in the entire sample, those with 'stronger' EI scores seemed to have more favourable leadership qualities. Finally, a recent review of the field (Akerjordet and Severinsson, 2010) concluded that more systematic research is needed into the role of EI in nurse leadership so we can investigate whether we can truly integrate EI and its implications into the education of nurses and other health and social care professionals.

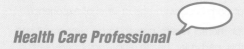

Health Care Professional

Male nurse

Breaking the stereotypes

I come from a traditional working-class town whose heavy industry has disappeared, otherwise I would have been expected to follow my Dad as an apprentice in skilled manual work. A few eyebrows were raised when I applied to become a 'male nurse', but

I took naturally to learning about mental health issues, which everyone has to deal with in some way or other. I've always had a knack for reading the signs in people's facial expressions, body language and the way they speak that indicate how they're feeling: happy, sad, angry, afraid, etc. In my line of work, it's important to detect these and understand why people behave in certain ways, or what they're likely to do, as all actions are based on thoughts and emotions, whether rational or not. Interpreting and understanding what's behind patients' actions is essential for working out how to respond and help them, and I'm good at that in and out of work. People may say that's normally a woman's talent, but then my girlfriend is much better than I at 'male' tasks such as DIY about our house. Differing talents, even the reverse of those expected, is what makes us a great team!

KEY POINTS

- EI is a person's ability to monitor their own emotions and the emotions of others correctly.
- Research does point towards EI being a good attribute to have in the health and social care field (most research has looked into nursing).
- More research is needed to see if it can help with leadership skills and also whether people can be 'taught' to increase their EI awareness.

EMPATHY
What is it?

Empathy is the ability to share someone else's feelings by imagining what it would be like to be in their situation. This may be because you have experienced something similar yourself. Therefore, it is more about *relating* with a patient in a health and social care setting. Remember that sympathy is just about acknowledging someone else's emotional issues and providing comfort based on that.

Empathy
The ability to share someone else's feelings by imagining what it would be like to be in their situation

Sympathy
Acknowledging someone else's emotional issues and providing comfort based on that

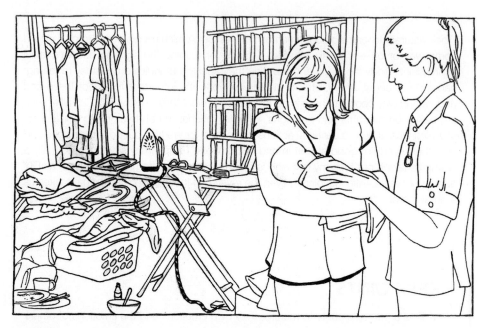

How will empathy with this new mother enable the health visitor to help her?

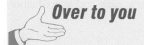 **Over to you**

You have a patient who needs to lose weight in order to improve their lifestyle and increase their chances of survival. They are really concerned that they cannot do it and will find it very difficult. How would you respond in (a) an empathic way and (b) a sympathetic way? One or two sentences is enough for this task.

How does empathy affect people who work in health and social care settings?

As noted in the study by Codier *et al.* (2010) earlier, empathy is part of EI and is therefore an important factor involved in health and social care professionals' working lives.

Recent research has been conducted to see if the amount of empathy declines as nurses' careers progress – so for example, do you they become 'immune' to this after being exposed to cases in real life hospitals etc. Nunes *et al.* (2011) investigated whether this was the case.

RESEARCH IN BRIEF

Nunes, P. *et al.* (2011) A study of empathy decline in students from five health disciplines during their first year of training

Aim: To examine if empathy declines in students from different health and social care disciplines 1 year into training.

Method: Over 350 students in the West Indies completed a questionnaire that measured empathy as soon as they started their training and then 1 year later. Students were training to be nurses, dentists, pharmacists, etc. The scores could be analyzed over time and then between the different health disciplines.

Results: Empathy scores were higher for females than males for all health disciplines. Nurses had the highest empathy scores on entry to training. All disciplines saw a decline in empathy when tested 1 year later and these were really marked for nurses and dentists.

Conclusions: It would appear that during the first year of training, nurses in particular have decreased empathy as measured by a questionnaire. The research team stated that some of this might be due to a shift from 'idealism to realism' (p. 12).

Reflective activity

Why do you think empathy can decline in students in health and social care professions? Think of at least three reasons why this may be the case (you can draw on personal experiences here).

However, Tavakol, Dennick and Tavakol (2011) examined the potential decline in empathy in medical students in the UK. They wanted to test if there were gender differences in empathy, whether empathy did decline throughout medical education and whether there was a difference between those ultimately intending people-oriented careers (e.g. family medicine etc.) compared to technology-oriented careers (e.g. radiology, surgery, etc.). Female medical students did score higher on empathy than male students. Those wanting to pursue the technology-oriented careers scored *lower* on empathy than those looking for people-oriented careers. However, there was no empathy decline in the sample of medical students. One drawback has to be noted though; this study was cross-sectional so each year group was tested at the same time. We must ask ourselves if the results would have been the same if they had followed the same students throughout their 5-year degree programme. What do you think?

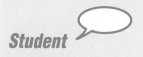

Student

A mature student

Does anyone understand?

I started my nursing course as a mature student, having worked intermittently as a Care Assistant until my youngest child had started school. I still work part-time some weekends out of financial necessity and find I do a lot of the family chores, as my husband works away from home, which doesn't always leave me much time or energy for study. My impression is that younger students, mentors and tutors don't understand my outside commitments and make no allowances.

I'm so glad that I have made good friends with students in the same situation; we encourage each other and hold our own study sessions to keep ourselves 'up to speed'.

A review of the empathy in health and social care field was conducted recently by Pedersen (2009). He examined over 200 studies that mentioned measuring empathy in health and social care professionals. He found that:

- Most of the studies did not even define what was meant by empathy yet they were supposed to be measuring it!

- Empathy was measured quantitatively in 171 studies (e.g. using rating scales via self-report questionnaires), using 38 different ways, so there appears to be no common way of measuring empathy via self-report questionnaires.

- Very few studies examined empathy using qualitative methods, so there is little in-depth analysis of why empathy could be important or whether a nurse feels empathy decline.

Pedersen's review casts doubt on findings of empathy decline as the measuring of it might not be clear or even correct.

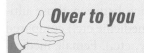

Over to you

It is recommended that you read Pedersen's review fully before reading any more research into empathy that has been performed since 2009 to see if more recent studies have got better at assessing empathy in health and social care settings. Find some studies from 2009 onwards and assess them using the findings from Pedersen (2009).

Another recent review also casts some doubt about empathy decline in health and social care professionals because the way it is measured may not be 'up to standard' (Yu and Kirk, 2009). They reviewed the literature from 1997–2007 and found 29 studies that had looked into empathy and nursing, using 20 different measuring tools. All of the measures had total scores between two and eight out of 14, meaning all scored quite low. It seems that more attention has to be paid to how empathy is measured in outcome studies and this review casts doubt on any current findings about aspects of EI, such as empathy decline as the measures used may not be robust.

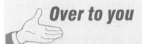

Over to you

How do you think empathy could be measured in health and social care research? Think about whether it can only be done via questionnaire.

Some health and social care researchers may try to explain the potential reduction in empathy as being a result of compassion fatigue.

KEY POINTS

- Empathy is the ability to share someone else's feelings by imagining what it would be like to be in their situation.

- Sympathy is about acknowledging someone else's emotional issues and providing comfort based on that.

- Based on research findings, empathy appears to differ within different fields of health and social care and it may decline over time.

- Research needs 'better' and more valid ways of measuring empathy to ensure findings can be applied to health and social care settings in the real world.

COMPASSION FATIGUE

What is it?

Compassion fatigue refers to when health and social care professionals experience both emotional and physical fatigue/tiredness due to an over-usage of empathy when dealing with patients' problems and conditions. The overuse of empathy 'builds up over time' so it is cumulative and can ultimately lead to

Compassion fatigue
When health and social care professionals experience both emotional and physical fatigue/tiredness due to an over-usage of empathy when dealing with patients' problems and conditions.

professional **burnout** when the person simply 'cannot face the emotional aspects linked to work'

Burnout
When the person simply 'cannot face the emotional aspects linked to work'

Coetzee and Klopper (2010) decided to come up with two separate definitions of compassion fatigue as they believed the literature was employing the term inconsistently. After reviewing the field and bringing together all the ideas relating to compassion fatigue they arrived at the following:

1 'Compassion fatigue is the final result of a progressive and cumulative process that is caused by prolonged, continuous and intense contact with patients, the use of self and exposure to stress. It evolves from a state of compassion discomfort, which if not effaced through adequate rest, leads to compassion stress that exceeds nurses' endurance levels and ultimately results in compassion fatigue. Compassion fatigue is a state where the compassionate energy that is expended by nurses has surpassed their restorative processes, with recovery power being lost' (p. 237).

2 'Compassion fatigue is the final result of a progressive and cumulative process that evolves from compassion stress after a period of unrelieved compassion discomfort, which is caused by prolonged, continuous and intense contact with patients, the use of self and exposure to stress. The manifestations increase in intensity with each progressive state, but the indicative signs of compassion fatigue are the physical effects of burnout, absence of energy and accident proneness, the emotional effects of breakdown, apathy and a desire to quit, the social effects of unresponsiveness, callousness and indifference towards patients, the spiritual effects of poor judgement and disinterest in introspection and the intellectual effect of disorderliness' (p. 239).

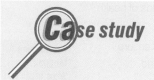

Case study

Burnout

For the past 20 years, Sister MacKenzie has been in charge of the nursing team in the very busy liver assessment and transplant unit of a large hospital in central Scotland.

The most common reason that patients are referred there is for cirrhosis due to prolonged, excessive intake of alcohol and forms of hepatitis related to intravenous self-administration of recreational drugs. Over the period of Sister Mackenzie's tenure, Scotland has steadily acquired the highest comparative mortality incidence of this condition among countries in Western Europe (Leon *et al.*, 2003).

Although immensely knowledgeable about her sphere of professional practice, Sister Mackenzie has become increasingly unable to offer clear or prompt advice to questions about patient care from more junior nursing staff, and has ceased to contribute to multidisciplinary team decisions, appearing to organize the roster to miss their meetings whenever possible. Her staff nurses try whenever possible to exclude her from medicine rounds, at which she is deemed 'a liability'.

Most of her time off-duty and holidays are spent helping to care for her increasingly dependent parents; she herself routinely retires to bed by 10.00 pm yet struggles to arise for morning shifts.

Secretly, she views the unit's clientele as deliberately inflicting their own health problems; many have ignored, despite promised 'good intentions', her repeated advice about the urgent need to reform their lifestyles. She now regards most of them as 'lost causes' and a burden on the taxpayer. Her attitude towards the unit's patients is not, however, as covert as she imagines.

Many of her current thoughts revolve around retirement, but that is not an imminently practical prospect.

1 How many of the features of compassion fatigue can you identify from the scenario above?

2 What steps might be taken to support Sister Mackenzie in her current situation?

3 Locate and read a published article concerning how health professionals relate to patients whose 'lifestyle choices' seem causally connected to their ill-health.

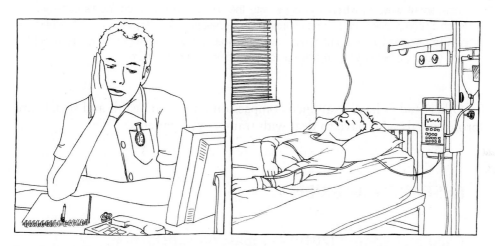

Compassion fatigue shows as lack of energy, and apathy as well as being accident prone, disorganized and having poor judgement.

How does it affect people who work in health and social care settings?

Aycock and Boyle (2009) were one of the first to propose the usage of the term compassion fatigue rather than burnout when referring to health and social care settings especially oncology nursing. They assessed the availability of resources available to nurses in such settings. Around 60 per cent of the hospitals surveyed had some sort of assistance programme, with 22 per cent having a counsellor or psychologist to help out nurses. Nearly half did not offer training for coping with this type of patient care and 82 per cent did not offer any 'off-site retreat to promote renewal' (p. 186). However, three hospitals had a yearly mandatory retreat for oncology nurses to cope with compassion fatigue. Potter *et al.* (2010) assessed the levels of compassion fatigue and burnout in oncology nurses in America. Over 150 health and social care providers completed a survey that measured aspects of their jobs like compassion fatigue. There was a significant relationship between compassion fatigue and work setting – those working in an inpatient setting were more at risk. Also, 44 per cent of those involved in this type of work setting have high risk of burnout. There was no effect of length of time practising in this speciality but those who had been working for 6-10 years in oncology had the highest percentage of high-risk burnout scores and the lowest compassion satisfaction scores (getting pleasure from doing your work effectively). Therefore, it would seem that nurses working in oncology are at risk of burnout via increased levels of compassion fatigue.

Reflective activity

Think about ways in which you cope with the different negative emotional demands (such as compassion) and compare them with a colleague. Are they the same? Are there new techniques you could now use based on what a colleague has told you that might help you cope better with negative emotional demands in the future?

Other studies have examined compassion fatigue in health and social care professionals who have to deal with traumatized patients.

RESEARCH IN BRIEF

Craig and Sprang (2010) Compassion satisfaction, compassion fatigue, and burnout in a national sample of trauma treatment therapists.

Aim: To examine levels of compassion fatigue, burnout and compassion satisfaction in health and social care professionals dealing with trauma.

Method: A total of 532 trauma specialists completed the same survey used in the Potter *et al.* (2010) study. Demographics and work status were also recorded. The sample consisted of 65 per cent females with an age range of 27–83 years. Virtually the entire sample (98 per cent) had patients on their 'casebooks' with post-traumatic stress disorder (PTSD). Participants had to rate how much they agreed/disagreed with each statement on the questionnaire. Examples of these statements included:

- Compassion satisfaction: 'I believe I can make a difference through my work' and 'I have happy thoughts and feelings about those I help and how I can help them'.

- Compassion fatigue: 'I think I may have been "infected" by the traumatic stress of those I help' and 'I feel as though I am experiencing the trauma of someone I have helped'.

- Burnout: 'Because of my work as a helper, I feel exhausted' and 'I feel "bogged down" by the system'.

Results:
For burnout the following factors appeared to be having a significant effect:

- burnout decreased with age
- those who had participated in special training on trauma had higher levels of burnout, which goes against 'common sense'
- the higher the number of PTSD patients in their caseload the more likely they were to burnout.

For compassion fatigue, the following factors had an effect:

- the higher the number of PTSD patients being looked after increased compassion fatigue
- those who had been exposed to evidence-based practice (using interventions that have been tried and tested to help overcome fatigue etc.) showed much less compassion fatigue.

Conclusion(s): It would appear that those working with traumatized patients do suffer from burnout and compassion fatigue like in other areas of health and social care. Exposure to more PTSD patients appears to have a negative effect on therapists but those who undergo help that is evidence-based and rigorous *may* combat the negative effects of this line of work in terms of reduced burnout and compassion fatigue but more research is needed based on the results of the special training in this study going against this idea.

Finally, Hooper *et al.* (2010) noted that emergency nurses appeared to have reduced levels of compassion satisfaction, intensive care nurses had a higher risk of burnout and oncology nurses were at a higher risk of compassion fatigue in their survey-based study. Also, for a recent review of the terminology of compassion fatigue and risk factors/prevention see Newell and MacNeil (2010).

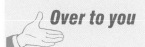

Over to you

You have been asked by your local health and social care provider to create a programme to help people who may be at high risk for burnout and/or have high levels of compassion fatigue. Design such a programme based on evidence and cover aspects like what you would cover, for how long you would have the programme for and how you would test its effectiveness.

KEY POINTS

- Compassion fatigue is cumulative and can lead to 'burn out'.
- Rigorous and evidence-based help may reduce compassion fatigue and burnout.
- Emergency, intensive care and oncology nurses are at the greater risk of compassion fatigue and burnout, with oncology nurses being at the highest risk.

CONCLUSIONS

As research indicates emotional intelligence is a good attribute to have in the health and social care field. More research is needed to see if it can help with leadership skills and to see whether people can be 'taught' to increase their EI awareness.

Effective evidence-based training and support to help health and social care professionals cope with the emotional demands of working with very ill people to help protect them from compassion fatigue and ultimately burnout.

RAPID RECAP

1 Outline how someone's personality might affect their work in a health and social care setting.

2 What is Emotional Intelligence?

3 What is the difference between empathy and sympathy? How can empathy affect workers in health and social care settings?

4 Can Compassion Fatigue affect workers in health and social care settings? Justify your answer using evidence.

If you have difficulty with any of the questions, read through this section again to refresh your understanding before moving on.

KEY REFERENCES

Other references are listed on the supporting website.

Craig, C.D. and Sprang, G. (2010) Compassion satisfaction, compassion fatigue, and burnout in a national sample of trauma treatment therapists. *Anxiety, Stress & Coping*, 23(3): 319–339.

Coetzee, S.K. and Klopper, H.C. (2010) Compassion fatigue within nursing practice: A concept analysis. *Nursing And Health Sciences*, 12: 235–243.

Leon, D.A., Morton, S., Cannegieter, S. and McKee, M. (2003) **Understanding the Health of** Scotland's Population in an International Context: a review of current approaches, knowledge And recommendations for new research directions, A report by the London School of Hygiene & Tropical Medicine, Commissioned and funded by the Public Health Institute of Scotland London: LSH&TM

Nunes, P., Williams, S., Bidyadhar, S. and Stevenson, K. (2011) A study of empathy decline in students from five health disciplines during their first year of training. *International Journal of Medical Education*, 2: 12–17

Pedersen, R. (2009) Empirical research on empathy in medicine – A critical review. *Patient Education And Counseling*, 76: 307–322.

Salovey, P. and Mayer, J. (1990) Emotional Intelligence. *Imagination, Cognition and Personality*, 9(3): 185–211

Steptoe, A. and Wardle, J. (2001) Locus of control and health behaviour revisited: a multivariate analysis of young adults from 18 countries. *British Journal of Psychology*, 92: 659–672.

van Dusseldorp, van Meijel and Derksen (2010) Emotional intelligence in mental health nurses. *Journal of Clinical Nursing*, 20: 555–562.

CHAPTER 4

SOCIAL INTERACTIONS IN THE HEALTH AND SOCIAL CARE SETTING

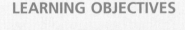

LEARNING OBJECTIVES

By the end of this chapter you should be able to:

- outline causes of aggression in people and describe research into aggression in health and social care settings

- explain ways in which aggression can be dealt with in health and social care settings

- describe what prejudice is and how it could develop in people

- outline theories of prejudice

- appreciate how health and social care professionals' own prejudices might affect them in health and social care settings

- outline ways to tackle prejudice and apply them to health and social care settings.

AGGRESSION

Theories on the causes of aggression

Biological explanations

Aggression
Any hostile or violent behaviour (physical or psychological) directed towards another person

Hormones have been linked to aggression. Testosterone is sometimes referred to as 'the male hormone' and increased levels have been linked to increased aggressive levels in humans. Carlson (1998) reviewed evidence for this in animal studies and reported that testosterone *organizes* and *activates* aggressive behaviours in non-humans. If immediately after birth, a rat, for example, is injected with testosterone it is *organizing* the rat to be aggressive later in life. However, this only actually happens if testosterone is injected when the treated rat is fully grown, which then *activates* aggressive behaviours. Rats that did not have the injection when fully grown showed lower levels of aggressive displays. That is, the early exposure to testosterone helped the development of testosterone-sensitive neural pathways, which were then used effectively later in life when exposed to more testosterone. In addition, the extra testosterone may make young male rats much more confrontational.

Frustration-aggression hypothesis

Dollard *et al.* (1939) proposed the link between frustration and aggression. In basic terms the more frustrated we get the more likely we are to become aggressive. The main cause of frustration is when we want to perform a certain behaviour and something or someone stops us from doing it. There are three factors involved:

1 The strength of the original drive. For example, if you are hungry at work and you are stopped from having lunch due to an 'emergency', you will be more frustrated if you were very hungry compared to being only slightly hungry.

2 How much the end behaviour has been thwarted. For example, if you only managed to eat half of your lunch on your break before being called back to work compared to just one bite then you would be less frustrated.

3 The number of frustrated responses. For example, you had your one bite of lunch, helped someone then had one more bite before being asked to help someone else, this would frustrate you more than just one interruption!

Social Learning (Bandura 1977)

This theory looks at the role of observation the act of watching someone's behaviour and imitation the act of repeating an observed behaviour in the development of aggression. This takes place over four stages:

1 Attention – the observer must pay attention to a role model (someone of a higher status and/or who has similar characteristics to the observer, for example, a role model or a character from the television). In this case, the role model would have to be someone who displays regular aggressive behaviour.

2 Retention – the observer must retain the aggressive act in their memory. This is the cognitive element of the theory, as the observer has to process the information they have witnessed.

3 Reproduction – the observer must feel that they are capable of imitating the aggressive act they have witnessed. Sometimes this can be very easy like kicking-out or be extreme like using a knife.

Observation
The act of watching someone's behaviour

Imitation
The act of repeating an observed behaviour

4 Motivation – the observer is more likely to reproduce the behaviour if they have experienced vicarious reinforcement. This is when the observer witnesses the role model getting rewarded for an aggressive act. This increases the probability that the observer will imitate that behaviour.

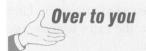

Over to you

Think about the motivation stage of Social Learning Theory. Consider an act of aggression you have witnessed and what rewards were given that you witnessed.

Research into aggression in health and social care settings

Magnavita and Hepniemi (2011) examined workplace violence and aggression against nursing students and nurses in Italy. After completing a range of questionnaires, it was discovered that 44 per cent of nurses and 34 per cent of nursing students reported having *at least one* physical or verbally aggressive encounter in their job. Nurses reported having more physical assaults and sexual harassments than nursing students, which may have been expected as they have had more exposure to health and social care work settings. However, there were marked differences in the sources of aggression. Nurses were more likely to have aggressive encounters with patients or their relatives, whereas nursing students were more likely to have aggressive encounters with colleagues, staff and teachers. In the period of 2010/11 to 2011/12 there was a slight rise of 3.3 per cent in total reported assaults on NHS staff from 57 830 in 2010/11 to 59 744 in 2011/12. Being on the receiving end of verbal aggression was strongly correlated with psychological problems. These latter findings were also reported by Fujishiro, Gee and de Castro (2011) in nurses in The Philippines. Those who reported more verbal assaults at work had poorer general health and work-related stress. Interestingly, 34 per cent of the sample reported having some form of verbal assault in the last 12 months (similar to the Italian figures above) but only 7 per cent had experienced a physical assault. Previous research in Italy (Zampieron *et al.*, 2010) had shown that up to 49 per cent of nurses had aggressive encounters at work (of which 82 per cent of these were verbal in nature). In this study, female nurses reported much higher levels of aggressive encounters and especially those who worked in emergency departments, geriatric units or psychiatric units. The majority of aggressors were either the patient or family and 66 per cent were male. Fifty-three per cent of the nurses did not seek help after their encounter. This appears to be common behaviour in health and social care professions. Could this be rectified with ways of dealing with aggression via training?

Dealing with Aggression

Reflective activity

Think about how you would cope with a patient who is being:

(a) verbally aggressive towards you

(b) is being physically aggressive towards you

(c) being verbally and physically aggressive towards you

(d) is being aggressive towards a work colleague in front of you.

Were your attempts all the same or should you tackle each one differently?

It may appear obvious but some form of training appears necessary for health and social care professionals to deal with aggressive behaviour within the workplace. Recently, Farrell, Shafiei and Salmon (2010) proposed a model for training staff in health and social care settings to deal with 'challenging behaviour' like verbal and physical aggression. The research team reviewed the literature from 1998–2008 to try to find examples of theoretically driven ideas for training health and social care staff so they could then amalgamate them into a Training Model. This model covers the following:

- The influence of the nurse/health and social care provider. This covers aspects like their values, emotional processes and their behavioural skills.
- The characteristics of the patient that may cause challenging behaviour.
- The features of the health and social care setting that might be influencing behaviour, such as its culture, current working practices and the physical environment.

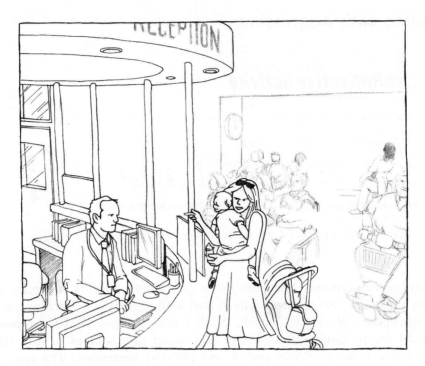

How would you deal with aggressive behaviour?

The model looks like this:

		Domains				
		Self			Other	Situation
		Values	**Emotion**	**Skills**		
		Value that learners attach to others (ranges from altruism to prejudice)	Emotions that affect learners' responses to others	Skills required for successful interpersonal interaction.	Factors That influence peoples' reactions to illness and care	How the cultural and physical environment shapes behaviour.
Levels	**Understand how challenging behaviour is influenced by...**	...one's values	...one's emotions	...one's repertoire of communication skills	... peoples' responses to illness and care	...the cultural and physical environment
	Apply this understanding to ...	...ensure that professionally appropriate values influence one's behaviour	...manage one's emotions in interactions	...acquire any new skills as needed	... work with the other's perspective	...manage the environment's influence on others' behaviour

Figure 4.1   The S$_{VES}$OS Model, where SOS stands for self, other and situation, S$_{VES}$ stands for self (Values, Emotions, Skills)

The research team wanted to show that there are many factors that contribute to challenging behaviour (and how we label it) so being able to deal with aggressive behaviour is not just a 'skill' we have to learn. Health and social care professionals need to be made aware of the following:

- How they label 'challenging behaviour' in certain types of patients (e.g. those with dementia or those who find communicating difficult and so get frustrated).

- Emotional reactions of staff towards potentially challenging behaviour like their own hostility or 'sadness' towards terminally ill patients who 'complain' as they want more pain relief.

- The environment in which they work – the research team quoted evidence that people with 'intellectual disability' reduced their level of challenging behaviour when moved from a ward to a community-based caring system. Lack of stimulation and even colour schemes on the wards have been related to boredom and frustration.

- Communication skills do require development in some health and social care professionals.

All of the five domains in the above model (Self Values, Self Emotion, Self Skills, Other and Situation) need to be covered, for training to be successful so that workers can effectively deal with challenging behaviour, like aggression.

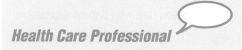

Health Care Professional

Assistant Practitioner

Diffusing tension in A&E

As an assistant practitioner in a busy Accident & Emergency Department, I encounter quite a lot of aggressive incidents; weekend nights are worst for this, and it's mostly the result of too much alcohol impairing people's judgement and lowering their inhibitions. Most commonly it's young males who become threatening, but mature people and females can also be challenging! The mass media can exaggerate reality; most of the time our team members can defuse angry patients by listening to their complaints and offering explanations. For instance, it's important to speak regularly to everyone personally, and attribute delays in their being 'seen' to the number of concurrent attendees, not to our deliberately ignoring anyone. Similarly, 'queue jumping' results from assessment of individual priority, our 'triaging' system.

If people are able to understand the reason for delays and are given a realistic estimated timescale, they are less likely to get uncontrollably frustrated.

Occasionally, communication skills aren't sufficient; our regular in-service updates provide us with techniques for managing incipient violence using de-escalation, break-away and containment methods; even then, the hospital always has security personnel available, plus police officers on site during predictably busy periods.

I have confidence in my own and my colleagues' ability to keep everyone safe in our A&E department, though there's seldom a dull moment here!

Hills (2008) had already assessed how aggression management training in particular had helped nurses in Australia. In his sample, over 76 per cent had experienced some form of aggression towards them in the previous 3 months. Around 40 per cent had not participated in any aggression management training or updated their training in the previous 5 years. The vast majority had low to medium perceived self-efficacy when dealing with aggressive patients. Hills stated that:

> *The finding that participation in aggression minimization training in the previous 5 years had only a very low or no significant impact on the frequency or type of patient aggression experienced in the previous 3 months, or on perceived self-efficacy in dealing with patient aggression, is concerning.'*
>
> *Hill (2008) (p. 28).*

Hopefully the new model from Farrell, Shafiei and Salomon (2010) can help to stop this trend and get health and social care professionals believing they can deal with patient aggression.

Reflective activity

What training opportunities are available to you to help you deal with patient aggression in your chosen health profession.

KEY POINTS

- There are biological, psychological and social factors that all play a role in aggressive behaviour shown in humans.
- Testosterone can cause humans to be aggressive. Frustration with daily events or prevention from completing tasks can also make us aggressive. Witnessing and then imitating aggressive acts could also make us aggressive.
- The amount of aggression shown by patients towards health and social care staff continues to rise across the world.
- There are new training methods for health and social care settings that can help professionals deal with this increased level of aggression seen in patients.

PREJUDICE

What is Prejudice?

The term prejudice, to prejudge someone based on little or no information, can be broken down into its component parts: pre and judge. Therefore, it is to prejudge somebody based on things like personality, occupation, sex, religion, etc. It is a thought or feeling you have (usually negative) against a person or a group of people. Quite a lot of people's prejudices are of other people whom they have never even met! These thoughts and feelings can sometimes affect our actual behaviour and this is when we use the term discrimination, which is used to describe how we act upon our prejudicial thoughts and feelings.

> *Over to you*
>
> Have a think about the profession you are currently training to become part of. What sorts of prejudiced thoughts and feelings may people have towards your profession and is there any evidence of discrimination towards it?

So, in essence, prejudice follows a CAB model as highlighted next, which could help us to understand what they are. CAB stands for Cognitive element, Affective element and Behavioural element.

> *Over to you*
>
> Someone you know has a prejudice towards students! Their cognitive element might involve thoughts like 'all students are lazy' whilst their affective element might involve feelings like anger and resentment. What might their behavioural element involve? Repeat this process for another prejudice that someone might have and see if there are any similarities and/or differences before reading on.

Development of Prejudice: Stereotyping

There are many different ideas about how we develop prejudices. One key element appears to be stereotyping. Horowitz and Bordens (1995) define it as 'a set of rigid beliefs, positive or negative, about the characteristics or attributes of a group' (p. 179). Therefore, we assume that people within a

Prejudice
To prejudge someone based on little or no information

Discrimination
How someone acts upon their prejudicial thoughts and feelings

Cognitive elements
The thoughts about the person or group of people that we have prejudices towards

Affective elements
The feelings we have towards the person or group of people we have prejudices towards

Behavioural elements
The actions we take as a result of the cognitive and affective elements towards the person or group of people we have prejudices about

Stereotyping
A set of rigid beliefs, positive or negative, about the characteristics or attributes of a group

group share a lot of commonalities even when in reality two people assigned to a 'group' can be very different indeed.

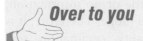

Over to you

Now, think about any similarities or differences you have with your closest friends on your course. Is it fair to group you by occupation, for example, 'occupational therapy students'?

Stereotypes can be positive (e.g. all nurses are caring and sympathetic) or negative (e.g. all students are lazy). Think back to the *Over to you* exercise earlier, how many of your answers were based on stereotypes? Stereotyping can be seen as being part of our Cognitive Toolbox (Horowitz and Bordens, 1995) that allows us to make judgements quickly about people in the world. It is a cognitive time-saver; think about how much time it would take to get to know the people you are stereotyping!

A recent study in Australia (Eley and Eley, 2011) reported that some of the stereotypical traits associated with the profession of nursing may well be true. Compared to an equivalent sample of GPs, a sample of Registered Nurses scored higher on measures of Novelty Seeking (things like 'seeks a challenge', 'is curious') and Reward Dependence (things like being 'sentimental and warm', 'seeking approval of others' and 'dedicated and attached to their patients'). These are 'typical' stereotypes that people have about nurses. In addition to this, Meadus and Twomey (2011) reported that male nurses still have trouble with people 'gender-stereotyping' them when training. They found that male nurses come across people who might say to them 'have you ever thought of becoming a doctor?' They also sometimes felt like they were an 'intruder in the profession' (p. 275) and many reported that even children, without any prompting from their parents would call them doctor rather than nurse. Finally, Gray (2010) discovered that in a group of nurses working in London, gender stereotypes were encountered quite regularly. He reported the following main finding:

> *General nursing was seen as feminine work that involved washing and close physical contact with the patient. Mental health nursing was viewed as being more masculine and the occupation of the majority of male nurses. Female nurses were seen as natural carers and emotional labourers of the patient's body. Male nurses in mental health sometimes had to deal with 'physical aggression', had to be 'physically stronger' and remedy disturbances of the patient's mind.*
>
> *Gray (2010)(p. 355).*

Many male nurses feel uncomfortable with the close physical and emotional contact with patients and being labelled as 'gay' and 'effeminate' were feared, especially if a male nurse wanted to pursue general nursing or midwifery.

The issue related to all of these stereotypes is that they can affect how people, like nurses, cope with the workplace in terms of potential discrimination from patients or experiencing negative situations involving people who hold these stereotypes. Harding (2007) studied the 'classic' stereotype that male nurses are gay. He reported that in reality, it is a minority of male nurses who are gay but that all male nurses are 'grouped' together under the same stereotype. One of the transcripts from Harding's interviews highlights this very clearly:

> A guy who had broken one of his legs needed a urinal and he rang the bell...and I remember a visitor, a guy, walked past and said to him, when he saw me with the bottle as I started to pull the curtains, "you'd better watch out for them, you know what they're like'.'
>
> Harding 2007, p. 639

Harding (2007) also noted that there were some interesting stereotypes that people held, especially that the general nurse is 'homosexual' if male but the male psychiatric nurse is most definitely 'heterosexual'. Harding noted that these ideas can easily prevent males entering the profession and may also explain retention issues in nurse training in New Zealand where the study took place.

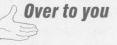

Over to you

Later on in this chapter we will look at ways to tackle prejudice. Before reading that section, have a think about ways in which you feel we could reduce the stereotyping and prejudice encountered by nurses in the Meadus, Gray and Harding studies you have just read about.

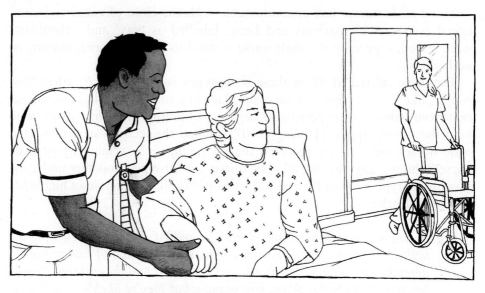

How would you cope if a patient showed prejudice against you?

Here is a case study about stereotyping, this time of a patient by a nurse.

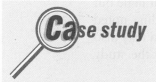

Dangerous assumptions

Joseph Jones is a youthful-looking 30 year-old with intellectual (learning) disabilities, who has been admitted to a surgical ward for a minor operation. None of the ward staff has had direct experience of looking after a 'mentally handicapped' patient, and concerns were immediately raised at the next shift handover about Joseph's potential dependency, inability to co-operate and challenging behaviour. Difficulties surfaced at the initial admission interview, when the nurse involved was rebuked by Joseph's mother for addressing questions to her rather than to her son; Joseph laughed long and hard at this.

Embarrassed by having underestimated the new patient's abilities, the nurse later left the menu selection card with a pen on Joseph's bedside table for him to complete; the following day no meal trays were delivered in the ward's trolley for Joseph, and the kitchen staff were adamant that his form had been returned entirely blank. Another nurse asked over the telephone for a selection that she assumed a child might enjoy, such as soup, cheese sandwiches and jelly and custard. Joseph refused any food that day. Soon it became clear that 'Joey', as the staff had renamed him, was unable to read or write.

His newly prescribed medications the next, pre-operative evening also met with refusal; the two nurses administering the round attempted in ever more strident tones to persuade him of the need to comply, and when one tried to pour liquid into his mouth, Joseph knocked it out of her hand, staining her immaculate uniform. The duty doctor was summoned, and ordered the nurses to administer a sedative to Joseph by intramuscular injection. When this was performed after minimal explanation, Joseph bellowed for some time and many of the other patients complained about the furore. Subsequently, Joseph was wheeled lying in his bed into a side-room, where the side-rails were raised and he was given firm medical instructions emphasized by close, fixed eye contact *not* to try and get up until the morning. At this point, he struck the doctor with the urinal that had been given to him 'in case of little accidents overnight'.

1 How closely does the scenario relate to the 'four stages' of the self-fulfilling prophecy?

2 How might the health professionals have improved their approach to meet Joseph's needs?

3 Read a publication that explains the particular needs of patients with learning disabilities and how these can be appropriately fulfilled by health and social care workers.

Theories of prejudice

There are many theories that psychologists have proposed that attempt to explain *why* people become prejudiced against others. We will look at some of the more popular ones.

Social Identity Theory

Tajfel and Turner (1979) produced one of the first psychological theories of prejudice development. The basis of the theory is centred around 'group membership' and how these can affect the way we think about the world, how we feel about the world and how we act in the world. There are three stages to their theory:

Social categorization is when we classify ourselves and others as being part of different social groups. You can be a member of more than one group, depending on things like your gender, occupation, hobbies, etc. These are called 'in-groups' (the group we immediately belong to) and 'out-groups' (the other groups around us).

Social identification is when we adopt an identity that is linked to the group we have categorized ourselves or others into. This is called **in-group favouritism** as we follow the group expectations when being part of that group. We may wear the same clothes (e.g. uniform or sports kit) and believe in the same things when we are behaving as part of that group. So, we take on the norms and attitudes of our in-group.

Social comparison is when we compare our group to other groups. We look favourably on members of our in-group and not so favourably towards an out-group to help boost our self-esteem. We begin to believe our group is better than the rest and this helps to boost our own self-esteem. We exaggerate the differences between groups whilst minimizing differences within our own group.

> **Social categorization**
> When we classify ourselves and others as being part of different social groups

> **Social identification**
> When we adopt an identity that is linked to the group we have categorized ourselves or others into

> **In-group favouritism**
> When we follow what is expected of when being part of that group

> **Social comparison**
> When we compare our group to other groups

Over to you

Make a list of all of the in-groups you currently feel 'proud' to be part of. Compare them with a friend who is also studying the same course as you are. Are there any similarities?

Therefore, we have many different in-groups depending on the social situation we find ourselves in.

This idea is based around 'labels' that we give people, for example 'aggressive', 'gay' or 'a nurse' – in the case of prejudice these may be the stereotypes we have already discussed. Once we have labelled someone we then 'expect' them to behave in a way that confirms our label. However, it is partly down to us and the way that we behave *towards* them, which makes them behave in a way that confirms our original belief – hence it is self-fulfilling!

The following highlights how **self-fulfilling prophecies** develop:

1 We give people a label (e.g. a stereotype), which means that we expect them to behave in a certain way.

2 We act in a way around this person that tries to confirm our label. Therefore, people are treated in a way based on the label given.

3 The person who is labelled reacts to this by behaving in a way that confirms the label. They act in a way that is 'expected of them' according to the label.

4 The behaviour from the labelled person fulfils expectations, which then completely confirm that label. And so the behaviour continues.

So, for example, you have a stereotype that a boss should be angry and aggressive. You are just late for a ward changeover with them and you 'just know they will be angry at you!' (even though they may not be, you have assumed this). You do not apologize because you have this idea that whatever you do they will be angry. This then makes them angry and you have confirmed to yourself that bosses are angry people. Totally self-fulfilling!

Self-fulfilling prophecy
When a belief we have causes itself to become true because of our actions towards others and the concept of labelling

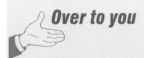

Over to you

Think about your profession and see if you can use *self-fulfilling prophecy* to explain why someone might have a prejudice against your profession using the four stages highlighted above. Does it work?

Attribution Theory

Over to you

Before you read this section, think about the following scenario. You arrive at work and immediately see one of your best friends/favourite colleagues walking towards you. You say 'good morning, how are you?' but they do not reply and in fact just walk straight past you! What are you left thinking?

There are many theories about how we try to find reasons for the causes of behaviour in people. We will focus on one called the fundamental attribution error. The idea of this error is that we tend to attribute the causes of someone's behaviour as being dispositional (within the person) rather than situational (looking at the environment as the cause). Therefore, we are much more likely to blame someone else's shortcomings for their behaviours rather than looking for other potential causes. This can help us to explain some prejudices in the following ways:

1 Western culture emphasizes the importance of individuals taking responsibility for their own actions and behaviours. Therefore, we may be prejudiced against heroin users as we see they 'bring it on themselves' rather than looking for environmental or social causes for their behaviour. This can then lead us to treat them differently as 'why should we help people who have brought on the problem themselves'. This, of course, can be an erroneous or not wholly valid belief on our part, which can lead to prejudice.

2 Perception of social situations – in perceptual psychology there is something called 'figure-ground effect'. That is, we focus our attention onto the object in the foreground and not on the background. Therefore, the person is the 'figure' in the foreground and the situation is the 'ground' (in this case the less obvious background) so we focus all of our attention on the figure to make sense of what is going on. This can then lead to prejudice against that 'figure'.

> **Fundamental attribution error** When the causes of someone's behaviour are attributed as being dispositional (within the person) rather than situational (looking at the environment as the cause)

Can health and social care professionals' own prejudices affect them in the workplace?

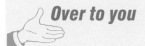

Over to you

In what way(s) may people's own prejudices affect how they deal with people in the workplace? Try to think of specific examples linked to your own profession.

RESEARCH IN BRIEF

Redpath *et al.* (2010) Health and social care professionals' attitudes towards traumatic brain injury (TBI).

Aim: To look into the attitudes of health and social care professionals towards people with traumatic brain injury and how this might affect helping behaviour.

Method: There were four groups of participants: first year trainee nurses, qualified nurses, first year trainee doctors and qualified doctors. They were randomly allocated to one of three causes of the brain injury (road traffic accident, drug use and aneurysm) which also had different 'levels' of blame. Therefore there were six possible scenarios (e.g. road traffic accident – no blame; drug use – blame, etc.). Each participant only read one story about the person with a brain injury. The participants also completed three questionnaires measuring helping behaviour and attitudes/prejudices. One measured potential prejudice towards people with brain injury using statements like 'Paul is responsible for his illness' and 'Paul deserves to die'. A second one measured the likelihood someone would interact with the person with questions like 'If you met Paul would you be willing to strike up a conversation with him?' The final questionnaire measured intention to help with questions like 'Given the busy nature of your work, is Paul someone you would perceive as low or high priority, in terms of staff time and NHS resources?' A total of 460 participants took part in this study.

Results: People who were to 'blame' for their own brain injury generated more prejudicial attitudes towards them irrespective of the cause (e.g. road traffic accident) from already qualified health professionals compared to the students. There was also an inverse relationship between level of prejudice and helping behaviour: those with higher levels of prejudice were less likely to show helping behaviour. This was only true for qualified health professionals.

Conclusion: 'Increased prejudicial attitudes of qualified staff are related to a decrease in intended helping behaviour, which has the potential to impact negatively on an individual's recovery post-injury' (p. 802).

Reflective activity

Why do you think the qualified health and social care professionals were more prejudiced and less likely to want to help than the ones still training?

There has been other research into the potential effects our own prejudices may have on how we deal with patients in the workplace. Poon and Tarrant (2008) examined prejudices towards patients with obesity. A sample of registered and trainee nurses completed the Fat Phobia Scale and the Attitudes Towards Obese Adult Patients scale. Registered nurses had higher levels of 'fat phobia' and more negative attitudes towards obese adults than trainee nurses. These attitudes included perceiving the obese people to like food a lot, being slow and unattractive. Over 50 per cent of the participants believed that obese patients should be forcibly started on a diet when they are admitted to hospital. The researchers were concerned about how these prejudices might affect how the patients were treated in hospital.

Frazer *et al.* (2011) examined prejudicial attitudes of nurses and other health and social care professionals towards patients with hepatitis C virus in the Republic of Ireland. It was concluded that younger nurses and those educated to degree level or above had the most positive attitudes and less prejudice towards patients with the hepatitis C virus, but a lot of the nurses wanted more education about the disease and how to care for people who have it. The research team concluded '*Negative attitudes can result in discriminatory experiences for persons with hepatitis C or at risk*' (p. 598).

Not all prejudice is overt, there are instances when our prejudices are unconscious but still affect our behaviour. This is called implicit prejudice. A recent study examined whether implicit prejudices towards drug users affected how they were treated. von Hippel, Brener and von Hippel (2008) got participants to complete a range of questionnaires to measure things like job satisfaction and implicit prejudice. They reported that there was a link between job dissatisfaction and intention to leave their job (which was to look after intravenous drug users). However, when they then examined the role of implicit prejudice, it appeared that it played a role in causing stress, which in turn had an effect on their intentions to quit their current job; implicit prejudice appeared to add to the stress of the job and make people more dissatisfied with it.

> **Implicit prejudice**
> When our prejudices are unconscious but still affect our behaviour

It is not always the prejudices of the nurses and health and social care workers that can affect workplace stress and satisfaction. Haber, Roby and High-George (2011) examined the experiences of health and social care workers in South Africa, who were caring for people living with HIV/AIDS (PLHA). It appeared that the PLHA health workers were discriminated against and felt a loss of status within the health and social care field as a result of their chosen career pathway. This resulted in many wanting to leave the profession. However, doctors and nurses appeared to want to leave PLHA work in South Africa and move elsewhere but stay in the health and social care profession. This shows that cultural perceptions and prejudice can have a marked affect on health and social care workers.

Ways to tackle Prejudice

Psychologists have proposed many ideas as to how to reduce prejudice in people. We will focus on just a few of these in this section. They include **challenging stereotypes with contact with the stereotyped group** and **establishing common in-groups**.

Challenging stereotypes

One way that has been successful is to challenge the stereotypes that people have about the groups they are prejudiced against.

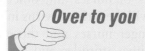

Over to you

Think about *how* you might challenge any negative stereotypes that people have about health and social care professionals? Are your ideas practical?

In order to do this, individuals from targeted groups have to be chosen carefully. They must be easily identifiable as part of an 'out-group' that has been stereotyped, but also be able to challenge stereotypes and show how people from the in-group have wrong assumptions.

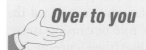

Over to you

Make a list of four different groups of people that have had prejudice aimed at them. Now, think about *who* could represent each group in order to challenge these stereotypes. Justify your choice(s).

Once the person or people are chosen that best represent the stereotyped 'out-group', the next stage can then be started: contact.

Contact with the stereotyped group

Allport (1954) proposed the idea that to reduce prejudice a member of an in-group needs to have direct contact with a member of an out-group who is of an equal status and where a mutual goal is needed to be reached. Desforges *et al.* (1991) took this idea further with a three stage-model:

1 Expectation. The person who knows that there is about to be some interaction between themselves and a stereotyped out-group member is going to expect someone similar to a typical member of that group.

2 Adjustment. If the meeting is on 'equal terms' then the whole process should be a positive one and the person with the prejudice should have a more positive impression of the other person.

3 Generalization. The positive experience was probably not expected (after all we are talking about prejudice!) but it should leave an impression that other members of the stereotyped group are the same and prejudice begins to be reduced.

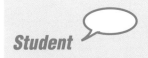

Student

Student nurse on a medical ward

Racism on the ward

Before my placement in a medical ward, I understood the importance of treating all people with respect and not making negative assumptions about them. I expected most of the patients to have accepted "multiculturalism" as a social reality, and was taken aback by a Mr Smith, who made increasingly loud and nasty comments about a person from a different ethnic group newly admitted to a neighbouring bed. I was really uncertain how to respond; should I ignore it, and hope the other patient wouldn't hear or be upset, or challenge each remark, and perhaps ruin the relationship I had formed with Mr Smith? Fortunately my mentor intervened, and Mr Smith was moved to an available side-room where the need for all patients to receive equal treatment free of harassment was forcefully explained to him. I later learned that Mr Smith had cancer, which had spread, to his brain, which might have contributed to his hostile attitude.'

RESEARCH IN BRIEF

Deacon (2011) How should nurses deal with patients' racism?

Aim: To observe and investigate how nurses deal with racism in acute mental health patients.

Method: This was a participant observation, so the researcher visited wards and simply observed what was going on. The observer simply fitted in with ward life and noted down occurrences of racism and how they were dealt with. Anything that was relevant to the study was noted down including, what the patients would say and how staff would deal with overt prejudice.

Results: There were many ways in which the nurses in the ward tried to understand why some patients would make racist remarks. One reason was as a consequence of their mental health issues. Some examples of the techniques that appeared to work included distracting the patient onto a different topic of conversation, politely asking patients to refrain from comment, ignoring them (so not to give them attention) or, as in some cases when things got really out of hand, sedatives to calm a patient who was also attempting physical abuse. All of the techniques had different degrees of success depending on the patient , so a 'one rule fits all' cannot work in a mental health unit. It looked like individual nurses in the study had a different technique that was most effective for them.

Conclusion: Deacon '...concluded that patients' racism cannot be managed by following simple, procedural rules but neither should it be managed "behind closed doors". A culture should be facilitated in which can one feel secure that colleagues and managers will take their concerns about personal racism extremely seriously and engage with, and value their contribution in working out just what to do in specific cases' (p. 493).

Reflective activity

How would you, as a midwife, tackle a pregnant woman who has been prejudiced towards a close colleague of yours? You may wish to find out what procedures your practice area already has in place for such events and see if any match up with the psychological techniques you have read about in this chapter like contact with the out-group or challenging stereotypes.

KEY POINTS

- Prejudices consist of a Cognitive, an Affective and a Behavioural component.
- Social Identity theory sees prejudice as a result of group membership (in groups are prejudiced towards outgroups via categorization, identification and comparison.
- A self-fulfilling prophecy may also cause prejudiced thoughts and actions. The label we give to people affect how we act towards them which may result in the target person confirming our original prejudiced label.
- The Fundamental Attribution Error may also cause prejudiced thoughts as we attribute the causes of another person's behaviour to dispositional factors rather than situational.
- Some prejudiced thoughts may be unconscious – this is called implicit prejudice.
- There are a number of ways that we can attempt to reduce prejudice like contact with a stereotyped group or challenging stereotypes.

CONCLUSION

Patients throughout the world are exhibiting increasingly aggressive behaviour towards health and social care staff and to help these professionals deal with this increased level of aggression seen in patients they should have the opportunity to experience the new training methods available.

There are different ways in which workplace prejudice may be tackled in health and social care settings. More research is obviously needed with relevant training to ensure that prejudicial thoughts and actions do not 'get in the way' of excellent health and social care.

RAPID RECAP

1 Identify two causes of aggression.

2 What are the four stages of Social Learning Theory?

3 How can prejudice affect workers in a health or social care setting?

4 Outline one way in which we can reduce prejudice.

If you have difficulty with any of the questions, read through the section again to refresh your understanding before moving on.

KEY REFERENCES

Other references are listed on the supporting website.

Deacon, M. (2011) How should nurses deal with patients personal racism? Learning from practice. *Journal of Psychiatric and Mental Health Nursing*, **18**: 493–500.

Gray, B. (2010) Emotional labour, gender and professional stereotypes of emotional and physical contact, and personal perspectives on the emotional labour of nursing. *Journal of Gender Studies*, **19**(4): 349–360.

Harding, T. (2007) The construction of men who are nurses as gay. *Journal of Advanced Nursing*, **60**(6): 636–644.

Redpath, S.J., Williams, W.H., Hanna, D., Linden, M.A., Yates, P. and Harris, A. (2010) Health and social care professionals' attitudes towards traumatic brain injury (TBI): The influence of profession, experience, aetiology and blame on prejudice towards survivors of brain injury. *Brain Injury*, **24**(6): 802–811.

CHAPTER 5

EXPLAINING AND CHANGING HEALTH BEHAVIOUR

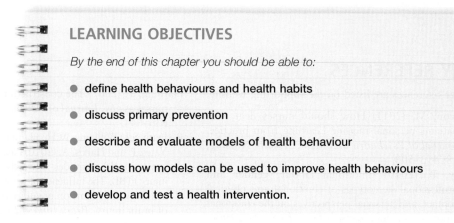

LEARNING OBJECTIVES

By the end of this chapter you should be able to:

- define health behaviours and health habits

- discuss primary prevention

- describe and evaluate models of health behaviour

- discuss how models can be used to improve health behaviours

- develop and test a health intervention.

Health behaviours
Actions that are beneficial or detrimental to health

Many service users and health and social care professionals alike acquire poor health behaviours, tending to do things that compromise health. This chapter explores why these behaviours arise and how people can be encouraged to avoid or limit health problems. The ideal solution is primary prevention, ensuring that healthy behaviours prevail over unhealthy ones.

Health behaviours can be explained in several different ways; the health belief model, the theory of planned behaviour and the transtheoretical model are discussed in detail. Successful health and social care requires not only an understanding of why people behave in unhealthy ways, but what can be done to overcome these problems. The theories discussed are considered with respect to their implications for health education. One way in which this knowledge is used is through health interventions. Examples are used to explore how health promotion can be used to raise awareness and change attitudes towards health issues and ultimately to change behaviour.

Primary prevention
Strategies that avoid risk and promote health in currently healthy individuals

HEALTH PROMOTION, HEALTH BEHAVIOUR AN HEALTH HABITS

Health promotion
Strategies employed to enhance public health

People tend to engage in behaviours that impair their health and fail to commit to activities that could protect or improve their health. Health promotion aims to enable people to gain control of, and therefore enhance, their health. This may be through lifestyle changes, such as taking exercise, eating a different diet or reducing alcohol consumption and through preventative practices such as breast and testicular self-examination and dental check-ups. Those activities that people do to maintain or improve their health are called health behaviours. People who engage in poor health behaviours not only compromise their health in the short term but may develop poor health habits, that is, they may acquire firmly established health-related behaviours that are detrimental. We begin to develop health habits at 11 or 12 years-old and they may become so automatic that we perform them without awareness.

> **Health habits**
> Behaviours relating to health that, over time, have become automatic and may be performed without awareness

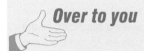

Over to you

Can you remember cleaning your teeth this morning? It's probably a health habit that is so automatic you don't recall doing it. Now consider your answers to the questions below about the seven health habits studied by Belloc and Breslow (1972). They asked almost 7000 Californians about the seven health habits listed below. Those with better health habits took fewer days off work and, when followed up almost 10 years later, had a lower mortality rate (Breslow and Enstrom, 1980). How would you score?

- How many hours sleep do you get?
- Do you smoke?
- How often do you eat breakfast?
- How many alcoholic drinks do you have on average per day?
- How often do you exercise?
- Do you eat between meals?
- Are you overweight?

Good health habits are important. They are particularly important for health and social care professionals, who are role models for the patients in their care and role models can change the behaviour of others when they are imitated.

RESEARCH IN BRIEF

Blake *et al.* (2011) 'Do as I say, but not as I do': Are next generation nurses role models for health?

Aim: To find out about the health behaviours and well-being of pre-registration nurses in an acute NHS teaching hospital in England.

Procedure: Pre-registration nurses were given a health and lifestyle questionnaire, which measured levels of physical activity, smoking and alcohol behaviour, dietary practices and general health.

Results: 325 nurses responded (50 per cent response rate) (aged 19-53 years, 96 per cent female). Of these, over half of these did not meet public health recommendations for physical activity and approximately one-third were classified as either overweight or obese. Just under one-fifth smoked and more than three-quarters did not eat five portions of fruit or vegetables per day. Two-thirds exceeded the recommended maximum daily alcohol intake. Physically inactive respondents were less likely to report good general health, good dietary practices and more sleep, and were more likely to report cigarette smoking and alcohol consumption than their active counterparts.

Conclusions: The health profile of pre-registration nurses is poor, and less active nurses tend to engage in other negative lifestyle behaviours. Despite delivering significant health education for patients, this knowledge does not necessarily transfer to nurses' own behaviour. There is therefore a need for health promotion interventions early in the career of nurses.

Primary prevention measures

Positive health behaviours:

- Eating a balanced diet
- Eating less fat, salt and cholesterol
- Eating more fruit and vegetables
- Regular dental check-ups
- Self-examination (breast/testicular)
- Taking exercise
- Keeping vaccinations current
- Practising safe sex
- Regular cervical smear test
- Wearing a seat belt

Avoidance of health-compromising behaviours:

- Stopping smoking
- Stopping drug misuse
- Reducing alcohol consumption
- Avoiding stress

PRIMARY PREVENTION

Primary prevention aims to prevent disease in currently healthy individuals by developing good health habits and discouraging poor ones. Two strategies logically follow from this approach to health. First, behaviour change can be used to encourage people to substitute good health behaviours for poor ones. For example interventions to help people to lose weight by altering their eating habits and exercise patterns. Secondly, programmes may aim to discourage people from ever developing poor health habits, for example, educational campaigns to dissuade teenagers from starting smoking or trying drugs. Prevention is clearly preferable but may be difficult to achieve because:

- The range of behaviours known to be threatening to health is limited – for example tobacco, opiates and cocaine have all, historically, been believed to be beneficial to health.

- Early intervention may be hindered – even school-based programmes will be too late to protect young people against poor health habits acquired in the home. For example, children of smokers are more likely to smoke than children of non-smokers.

- The cognitive limitations of children younger than school-age may prevent full comprehension of the need for health behaviours.

- Developing successful strategies to prevent the acquisition of poor health habits depends on understanding this process but our knowledge of the development of such processes is poor.

- During the time when people acquire health-compromising behaviours they fail to recognize or accept the long-term threat and therefore lack any incentive to avoid the behaviour.

- Although knowledge and motivation are essential to changing behaviour, just providing information, or scaring people, does not necessarily prevent unhealthy behaviour.

RESEARCH IN BRIEF

Janis and Feshbach (1953) Effects of fear-arousing communications

Aim: To test whether fear is an effective motive to induce a change in health behaviour.

Procedure: Three 15-minute films were made of illustrated lectures presenting information about the dangers of poor oral hygiene. The recordings differed in their capacity to elicit fear:

- Strong: Focused on pain (e.g. from tooth decay) and other risks such as blindness and cancer and used photographs of decayed mouths.

- Minimal: Used diagrams and X-rays, avoided serious consequences other than decayed teeth and cavities.

- Moderate: Created an intermediate level of fear.

Each film was shown to a group of students and a fourth group saw no film. Those students who saw the films were asked how they felt immediately afterwards and completed questionnaires about their dental hygiene 1 week before and 1 week after viewing the film.

Findings: The strong fear appeal film created the greatest immediate concern and participants expressed greater motivation to look after their teeth. It also aroused the most interest but was rated negatively as it was unpleasant. After 1 week, however, the high fear arousal group could remember less information and the minimal fear group demonstrated the greatest change in behaviour, with 36 per cent (compared to 8 per cent of the strong fear appeal group) reporting improved oral hygiene habits.

Conclusion: Although fear appeals to generate strong emotional responses, these do not necessarily translate into changes in health behaviours such as dental hygiene. The fear elicited by such strong communications does not motivate health behaviour but results in individuals ignoring the problem or minimizing the importance of the threat as a result of their fear.

Health Care Professional

School Counsellor

Altering children's eating behaviours

Children are naturally curious and they like to try new things; although they can be cautious, particularly if someone they trust has told them that something tastes horrible. Having a positive attitude and using small non-edible rewards can help to shape children's dietary habits. But enabling children to make significant lasting dietary changes relies on co-operation from their family and carers. As a school counsellor I know this can be a challenge in itself as it is hard to find ways to effectively communicate with them particularly when the children come from such different backgrounds and I have so little contact with their parents.

NUTRITION

Health behaviours relating to nutrition most obviously include weight control but also relate to healthy eating in terms of the provision of sufficient and appropriate nutrients. The NHS report on Obesity, physical activity and diet (2012) found that 26 per cent of adults in England would be classified as clinically obese (with a Body Mass Index of 30kg/m^2 or more). In addition, 17 per cent of boys and 15 per cent of girls (aged 2 to 15) were classed as obese. Although lower than in 2004, it is still higher than in 1995 (when the figures were 11 per cent and 12 per cent, respectively). The additional demands which such trends place on health services account for the interest which governments show in promoting healthy eating habits. Chronically obese people are at greater risk from problems, such as heart conditions and diabetes than non-overweight people.

RESEARCH IN BRIEF

Horne et al (2010) Increasing pre-school children's consumption of fruit and vegetables: A modelling and rewards intervention.

Aim: To test the use of modelling and rewards to increase pre-school children's consumption of fruit and vegetables.

Procedure: This was a field experiment in a nursery, using a repeated measures design. Rewards for eating healthy food types were manipulated (the IV) and changes in consumption of eight fruit and eight vegetables, used in four sets (see Table 5.1) were measured (the DV). The rewards were stickers to wear and bricks from a construction set to collect. Modelling was achieved by showing the children videos of two characters 'Jess and Jarvis' who enthusiastically ate each food, naming it and giving it a label as a fruit or a vegetable and encouraged the children to 'eat them up to be big and strong'. Before each intervention phase there was a baseline test during which the children were offered a food set each day, at snacktime and lunchtime but without rewards for eating these foods. During the intervention phases, new food sets were offered, alternating rewards for eating ether fruit or vegetables. Rewards were given only at snacktime, and although both fruit and vegetables were offered, rewards were only given for one or the other.

Results: The interventions produced large and significant increases in target fruit and vegetable consumption and smaller, but also significant, increases for the paired, opposite category, non-target foods (e.g. the fruit on offer when a vegetable was rewarded). After each intervention there was also an increase in within-category generalization, i.e. the rewards for one vegetable increased consumption of other, non-rewarded vegetables. In addition, these increases generalized strongly from snacktime (when they were rewarded) to lunchtime, when they were not. Finally, the increases in fruit and vegetable consumption were maintained at 6 months after the rewards were stopped.

Table 5.1 The 16 experimental foods and the configuration of each food set presented in the study		
Food set	**Fruit pair**	**Vegetables pair**
1	Dragon fruit + mango (non-target fruit)	Green beans + baby sweetcorn (target vegetables)
2	Kiwi fruit + pawpaw (target fruit)	Baby carrots + courgette (non-target vegetables)
3	Star fruit + sharon fruit (target fruit)	Cucumber + yam (non-target vegetables)
4	Water melon + prune (non-target fruit)	Swede + mangetout (target vegetables)

Conclusion: These findings contradict the idea that providing rewards undermines any intrinsic motivation to eat healthy foods, instead demonstrating that a combination of modelling and rewards can produce lasting change in young children. This is important as such early interventions could help to establish a liking for a wide range of fresh fruit and vegetables, which should last into adulthood and help to counteract exposure to pressures from society, which tend to lead to obesity.

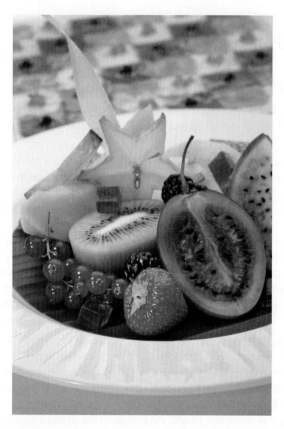

Eat fruit now, enjoy fruit later. Can childhood health promotion improve adult lifestyle choices?

In many parts of the world food is in short supply; malnutrition and starvation are appallingly common. In stark contrast, the difficulties for inhabitants of developed countries with regard to nutrition are, most significantly, weight control, although eating disorders and poor diet are also problematic. Humans have evolved to attend to the nutritional needs of active hunter-gatherers so are highly motivated to consume high-calorie foods. As a result people prefer the taste of fatty and sugary foods even though they are probably unnecessary in terms of energy output.

The task for psychology is not simply to understand the desire to overeat but to identify effective ways to control eating. This topic therefore provides us with the opportunity to look at a range of different explanations for health behaviours.

Psychological explanations of health behaviours relating to food

Lay beliefs suggest that there are biologically determined desires for food, like the 'food cravings' of premenstrual and pregnant women. Other eating habits are acquired; we might learn not to eat raspberry ice cream because we were once sick after eating some and – rightly or wrongly – formed an association between the two. Finally, beliefs about eating may be cultural. 'Spinach is good for the blood' and 'Carrots help you see in the dark' are two such guiding principles (each with a measure of biological foundation). So, health habits such as eating may be governed by three factors:

- Biology
- Learning
- Culture

To what extent is each of these determinants of our health behaviour important?

Biological explanations

An evolutionary explanation, as proposed at the beginning of this section, can explain for the tendency of people to overeat. Not everyone, however, does so. Differences between people may be accounted for by variation in metabolic rate, with obese people tending to have lower rates, utilizing energy from food more efficiently and converting surplus intake into fat. Evidence from twin studies suggests that there are inherited components to both basal metabolic rate and the storage of excess energy as fatty rather than lean tissue (Bouchard *et al.*, 1990). This, however, can only account for how excess food is utilized, not how much is consumed. This must be controlled by other factors.

Homeostatic theories suggest that our bodies have biological systems that monitor and adjust some aspect of our physiology, such as blood glucose (glycostatic theory), blood fat (lipostatic theory) or weight (set point theory). Each suggests that biological processes, such as hunger, metabolic rate and the laying down of fat, are controlled to maintain the particular variable around an optimum.

In set point theory (Brownwell and Wadden, 1992) the hypothalamus (a region of the brain) determines a bodyweight that the individual will maintain independently of moderate changes in food intake. Each individual's weight is 'set' at a particular point. So, when an individual eats a little more than they need to for weight maintenance, their metabolic rate rises, energy is used more quickly. Conversely, if they eat too little, the body responds with increased efficiency, lowering the rate at which energy is used. As a result, small increases or decreases in food consumption make little difference to long-term weight. This accounts for the failure of crash diets – in the absence of sufficient food, the body may simply conserve energy by lowering the metabolic rate so food is 'burned' more slowly. Experimental studies of systematic starvation and over eating support this theory, with weight change away from the set point being harder to achieve than the return, although there is also a tendency for some individuals to settle above their previous standard weight in either case, suggesting that the internal optimum may be affected by other factors.

Biological determinants of weight, such as metabolic rate and levels of fat cells, may have some genetic contribution, as evidenced by adopted children showing a closer match to the weight of their biological than adoptive parents and the similarity in weight between twins even when reared apart (Stunkard, 1988). Such findings do not suggest that the environment is unimportant. Indeed, even family trends may be explained by environmental rather than genetic factors. Mason (1970) found that 44 per cent of the dogs owned by obese people were also obese, compared to only 25 per cent of dogs with owners of normal weight!

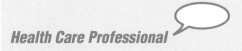

Health Care Professional

Dietician

Why some people have difficulty losing weight
'I work with many clients who find it hard to lose weight, to try to change their behaviour patterns. Very often they find it hard to lose weight *not* because they don't want to but often because they just find it really difficult. Many are on low incomes and find food with low nutritional value inexpensive and tasty – they say fresh fruit and vegetables cost more and don't taste as nice – while some who are struggling with their circumstances see food as reward, just a little treat to lift their mood. Often patients feel that because their parents were overweight it's inevitable that they will be too and will describe their families as big boned or having a low metabolism. Convincing people that they can do it by changing their behaviour patterns can take a significant amount of persuasion and considerable support but it's worth it.'

Behaviourist explanations

Learning theories can explain the acquisition of health behaviours. For example, the acquisition of 'comfort eating' may be explained using classical conditioning. Chocolate (unconditioned stimulus) tastes nice so makes us feel good (unconditioned response). In a situation where we are unhappy (neutral stimulus) we can experience an elevation in mood (unconditioned response) by eating chocolate (i.e. pairing the neutral stimulus and unconditioned stimulus), thus we learn to cheer ourselves up with food (conditioned response).

In operant conditioning, the frequency of a behaviour is affected by its consequences (reinforcers and punishers). Unhealthy food-related behaviours are often rewarding – chips and chocolate taste nice – thus they are positively reinforcing and performed more often. Whilst such behaviours do have unpleasant consequences on health (e.g. rotting teeth or damaging the heart) their effects are delayed so are ineffective as punishment.

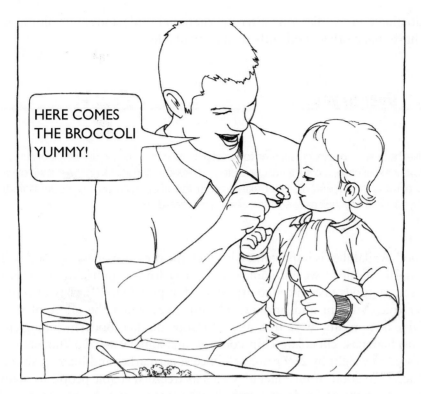

Children acquire good (or bad) health behaviours by imitating the behaviour of adults.

Social learning theory suggests that behaviours can be acquired by watching and imitating the actions of others. Thus we may like sweets because we see other children enjoying them but dislike vegetables if our siblings protest about eating them. Parents are also powerful models for the amount and types of food that children learn to enjoy. Messages from the media, such as television programmes and advertisements may also provide important role modelling. For example, Coon *et al.* (2001) compared children from families in which the television was on often versus on rarely, during meals times. Children from families who tended to watch television during meals ate more meat, pizza and salty snacks and less fruit, vegetables and juices. These differences persisted even when other factors, such as socioeconomic group, were controlled for. Similarly, Halford *et al.* (2011) experimentally controlled the exposure of 93 children to television adverts for either food or non-food items. After each type of advert, the children's consumption of a range of food was measured. Viewing the food adverts significantly increased total food consumption (see also Horne *et al.*, 2010).

Cultural explanations

Culture can account for some differences in food-related behaviour, including constraints, such as those imposed by Ramadan or Lent, and expectations, such as the consumption of rich foods for celebrations. In addition, cultural preferences may guide choices. For example, traditional foods may continue to predominate in the diet long after international trade and multicultural societies have made other foodstuffs readily available.

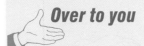

Over to you

Use the Internet or other resources to investigate food preferences of a range of cultures. In your experience, are such cultural dietary differences considered in the menus offered to patients in hospital? To what extent could this affect recovery? Consider both the physical and psychological effects of eating an altered diet.

Food availability is important. Although the presence of excess food will not necessarily result in weight gain, variety may lead to unhealthy choice: fatty and sugary foods taste nicer so are selected in preference. Variety also plays a direct role. Sclafani and Springer (1976) investigated the effect of a wide, variable diet on rats. With free access to 'supermarket foods' including cheese, salami, bananas, chocolate chip cookies, marshmallows and chocolate, they increased in weight by 269 per cent! Since supermarket and Internet shopping, and access to good storage facilities such as freezers, enable people to maintain a huge diversity of foods at home, healthy eating may be compromised by the powerful effect of novelty on satiation. Conversely, this illustrates the importance of offering patients who need to gain weight a varied diet.

KEY POINTS

Biological

- People are powerfully motivated by the taste of food, especially sweet and fat-rich flavours.
- Weight control programmes need to be tailored to individuals to combat the effect of different set points.

Behaviourist

- There is a need to counter-condition or unlearn associations that have been built up between unhealthy food and positive emotions or comfort.
- Healthy food must be perceived to be as rewarding as unhealthy food.
- Reinforcements are less effective if they are not immediate.
- Role models must exhibit positive behaviours towards healthy but not unhealthy foods.

Cultural

- Children's food choices are affected by advertising and this is not necessarily countered by adults' shopping behaviour.
- Cultural differences in eating habits may mean that different health issues arise within different cultural groups.

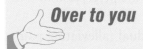

Over to you

Use biological, behaviourist or cultural explanations to account for the following food-related differences in behaviour:

- A child who is bullied in the lunch queue eats the vegetarian option in order to avoid his classmates, although he eats meat at home – later in life he doesn't like eating meat in restaurants.
- Two people of the same height and gender who eat identical diets and take the same exercise are not the same weight.
- Advertisements for chocolate often use images suggesting sex appeal.
- A family that encourages 'finishing everything on your plate' regardless of whether or not you are hungry finds that the children grow into adults who are indiscriminate eaters.
- Parents who tend to overeat have children who also overeat.

EXPLAINING HEALTH BEHAVIOUR
The health belief model

The health belief model (HBM) is a cognitive model that attempts to explain health behaviours by considering the variables that affect an individual's decision-making in relation to health-protective and health-compromising behaviours. It was originally proposed by Hochbaum (1958) and has been adapted several times (e.g. Rosenstock, 1966 and Strecher *et al.*, 1997).

> **Cognitive**
> Relating to attention, perception, thinking, reasoning or memory

The HBM identifies five core beliefs. These are:

- **Perceived vulnerability** – the individual's assessment of the risk that they will be affected by the condition (i.e. susceptibility).
- **Perceived seriousness** – the individual's assessment of how bad the effect will be if they are affected (i.e. severity).

Together, perceived vulnerability and seriousness determine the individual's perception of the threat posed by the disease. So, for example, a person who is asthmatic may recognize that this is a lethal condition (high perceived seriousness) but believe that because they don't get breathless during exercise they do not need to be concerned (low vulnerability). Where some threat exists, the individual must determine the extent to which engaging in a particular health behaviour will protect them. This is a balance between barriers and benefits.

- **Perceived barriers** – aspects of the situation that disincline the individual to take action. These may be financial (cost of prescriptions), situational (living a long way from a hospital) or social (not wanting to inconvenience other people by being off work). Time, effort and the perception of obstacles would also act as barriers.

- **Perceived benefits** – possible gains for the individual (alleviating pain or anxiety, improving health or reducing health risks).

Together, the perceived barriers and benefits present the individual with a cost–benefit analysis. For example, Abraham *et al.* (1992) studied Scottish teenagers, who were well aware of the seriousness of the risk of HIV infection, their vulnerability to it and the benefits gained by using condoms. However, condom use was prevented because the perceived barrier of costs, including loss of pleasure, awkwardness of use and anticipated conflict with their partner exceeded the perceived benefits of avoiding infection.

- **Cues to action** – for an individual to exhibit a health behaviour, even when the cost–benefit analysis judges it to be necessary, a cue to action is needed, that is, an immediate trigger to initiate the appropriate behaviour. This may be internal or external. For example, a patient may believe that they should stop smoking because it is a serious threat to their health, recognize their vulnerability and know that stopping would be advantageous. However, they may only do so on developing severe chest pains (internal cue) or if a relative dies of lung cancer (external cue).

The five core beliefs of the HBM should predict the likelihood that a particular health behaviour will arise in a given situation. Consider an example of a stressed individual with a high cholesterol level who believes that changing their eating habits to reduce their fat intake is going to reduce their risk of dying of a heart attack. They are more likely to persevere with the diet despite disliking it than a person who holds the belief that the fuss about cholesterol levels is all hype (low perceived seriousness) or that no-one in their family has heart problems so they are not at risk (low vulnerability).

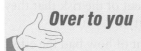

Over to you

Taking the example of someone who is obese and at risk from heart disease, identify the following statements relating to health beliefs and decide which person would be likely to embark on health-protective behaviours:

Patient A

- 'My chances of having a heart attack are low.'
- 'I don't want to turn into a jogging-junkie.'
- 'Exercising cuts down the risk of a heart attack but even sporty people still have them.'
- 'People who have heart attacks generally recover and go back to work.'

Patient B

- 'Heart attacks kill people.'
- I feel ready to start exercising more.'
- 'My neighbour had a heart attack and he was younger than me.'
- 'I guess that being stressed increases my chances of having a heart attack.'
- 'Getting fit will make me more attractive too.'

Evidence indicating that knowledge is important in bringing about appropriate health behaviours suggests that the provision of health information is worthwhile. Rimer *et al.* (1991) found that women who had more knowledge about breast cancer were more likely to have regular mammograms.

However, more information is not always beneficial. The Internet has made an enormous amount of health information available to patients despite the popular representation of the Internet as a reliable source of information, much of it is worryingly inaccurate. Matthews *et al.* (2003), in a survey of Internet sites about alternative therapies for cancer, found that, for two of the therapies considered, over 90 per cent of the websites surveyed contained incorrect information. Furthermore, ready access to information about health problems may increase anxiety rather than reducing it.

At least some uses of the Internet are, however, beneficial; Winzelberg *et al.* (2000) successfully used the Internet to deliver a health programme designed to reduce women's dissatisfaction with their body image.

Using the health belief model

The health belief model can be used to interpret behaviour in a number of contexts, for example to understand why people make use of or ignore disease prevention schemes and screening tests. Haefner and Kirscht (1970) found that people were more likely to use disease prevention measures and attend health screening services, including physical examinations and X-rays, if they were exposed to interventions that stressed vulnerability and the effectiveness of the particular health behaviour in combating the risk. Thus, the HBM cannot only help us to understand health behaviours but may provide a means to improve people's health.

Making use of disease prevention

Schemes for disease prevention include immunization, self-examination (of the breasts or testicles) and effective tooth brushing and flossing. The reason for encouraging people to engage in preventative measures is clear; it reduces health risks and early detection makes treatment easier.

Immunization is effective against diseases such as whooping cough (pertussis), measles, mumps and rubella (MMR) and many more. The

Immunization
Protection against disease by administering a vaccine to individuals before the infectious agent has been encountered

recent outbreak of measles in Wales has been speculatively attributed to the negative press coverage given to the MMR vaccination following the publication of Andrew Wakefield's now discredited research linking the vaccine to autism (Wakefield, 1988). McCartney reports that from 1997 a South Wales local newspaper published 26 articles questioning the safety of the vaccine. It is possible that these adverse media reports may have deterred parents from vaccinating their children, as vaccination rates did fall (although the newspaper did not ever say that parents should not immunize their children). These observations, if correct, would again suggest that the perceived benefits of vaccination do not outweigh the perceived barriers.

Murray and McMillan (1993) investigated the effectiveness of the HBM as a predictor of breast self-examination. A sample of 391 women completed questionnaires about their health behaviours, including the frequency of breast self-examination (BSE), and rated items reflecting their health beliefs, such as: 'My chances of getting cancer are great' (susceptibility), 'I am afraid to even think about cancer' (seriousness), 'If cancer is detected early it can be successfully treated' (benefits) and 'I just don't like doctors or hospitals' (barriers). They also provided information relating to their knowledge about cancer, their confidence in performing self-examination and whether any family member had ever had cancer.

The findings showed that breast self-examination was related to many variables, including knowledge and perceived benefits. Demographic variables such as age and social class also affected participation: young professional women were more likely to use BSE. However, some variables that are not considered by the health belief model were also important. The best predictor of appropriate action in this context was **self-efficacy**. Women who were more confident about carrying out breast self-examination were more likely to do so. This evidence suggests that health promotion should aim to improve confidence in the ability and to provide opportunities to practise the skill.

Self-efficacy
The extent to which an individual believes they can perform a particular behaviour adequately

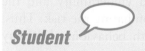

Student

Student nurse in a Day Care Unit

Both anxiety and information are important factors in determining health behaviour

'I got some leaflets from the health education centre about testicular self-examination and I asked to put them around the ward. One health and social carer said that they thought it would frighten the patients, raising their feelings of being at risk. From my learning in college about health belief models I think the availability of leaflets does not necessarily raise anxiety.'

Making use of screening tests

Screening tests include cervical smear tests for women, ultrasound scanning, amniocentesis and X-rays. As with disease prevention measures, screening enables health and social care professionals to detect diseases early and treat them more effectively. Participation in these health behaviours can be predicted, and appropriate directions for health promotion ascertained, using the health belief model.

Murray and McMillan (1993) investigated the power of the HBM to predict attendance at cervical cancer screening tests. The women were asked how many previous tests they had been for and why (e.g. doctor suggested it or routine postnatal check-up). When compared to measures of health beliefs, it was found that cervical smear testing (like breast self-examination) was related to knowledge and perceived benefits. However, the best predictor was 'barriers'. In other words, the women were more likely to have smear tests if they perceived little threat from the health service, the examination itself or the result. This suggests that attendance at smear testing could be improved by education to reduce the anxiety experienced by women about the investigation.

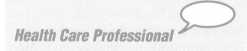

Health Care Professional

Practice nurses

Health Belief Model
Julie and Louise are practice nurses and talk about the time after the celebrity Jade Goody died from cervical cancer. We had hundreds of young girls coming forward for cervical screening tests even if they had not been before or had missed their appointment. The young women suddenly realized it was a disease that could affect them and that cervical cancer is a very serious illness. Although the test might be uncomfortable, knowing that if they had it would help them get treatment for their illness and prevent them losing their lives. Whilst Jade's death was a tragedy, it became a real "cue to action" for many women.'

Despite the evidence for the HBM, there are a number of criticisms. Health behaviours are affected by the factors proposed, but non-health-related motives, for example a desire to look good, are also important, e.g. to diet. Such variables cannot readily be taken into account by the HBM. Self-efficacy also matters; an individual may feel vulnerable and perceive benefits to changing their behaviour but without self-belief, they are unlikely to try. Korpershoek et al. (2011) conducted a review exploring the role of self-efficacy in the recovery of stroke victims. They found that higher self-efficacy was associated with better functioning in terms of activities of daily living and mobility, and a higher quality of life. It was also linked to lower depression.

Another important factor that the HBM cannot account for because it is a cognitive model, is the influence of emotions. An individual may fail to attend an appointment for a vaccination, even when they hold appropriate beliefs, because they have a phobia about needles – but this emotional component would not be explained by the HBM. The findings of Harvey and Lawson (2009) suggest that for diabetics, emotional factors are better predictors of adherence to advice for self-management than the variables considered by the HBM.

The theory of planned behaviour

Ajzen (1985, 1991) based the theory of planned behaviour (TPB), Figure 5.1, on an earlier idea, the theory of reasoned action. Like the health belief model, these are cognitive models, i.e. focus on the decision-making process of the individual. The TPB proposes that actions such as health behaviours are determined by a combination of behavioural intention (deciding to achieve a goal) and perceived behavioural control (believing that you can or cannot perform a behaviour).

So, consider the example of someone who wants to give up smoking, the two factors can be distinguished: first, wanting to be a non-smoker (behavioural intention), perhaps to avoid feeling excluded by non-smoking friends, and second, believing that you can achieve the goal (perceived behavioural control), for example feeling that you have the strength to over-come the unpleasant effects of nicotine withdrawal. Schifter and Ajzen (1985) illustrate the role of both factors in their study of weight loss in female students. Individuals who both expressed the intention to lose weight and perceived that they would be able to limit their calorie intake over the 6 weeks of the study lost more weight. This shows that intention only predicts healthy behaviour when perceived behavioural control is high.

Behavioural intention itself may be determined by **attitude** (which is affected in turn by knowledge) and by **subjective norms** arising from our beliefs and inclination to comply with these values. There are two components to sub-jective norms; normative beliefs about how others expect us to behave and motivation to comply. Considering the smoker again, they may believe that smoking is damaging to the lungs and heart, and may value health and fitness, resulting in an attitude that will make them more likely to give up. In this respect TPB resembles the health belief model as it considers the role of beliefs in affecting behaviour. The smoker may also consider subjective norms such as how their family feels about smoking (normative beliefs) and may be compelled to follow their example or advice (motivation to comply).

The relationship between behavioural intention and action has been sup-ported empirically. Research has successfully applied TPB to a range of health behaviours, including smoking (Norman and Tedeschi, 1989), weight loss (Schifter and Ajzen, 1985) and breast cancer detection (Montano and Taplin, 1991). Eagly and Chaiken (1993) report successful application of the model to other health behaviours such as blood donation, contraception, consumption of junk food, dental hygiene, having an abortion and smoking cannabis.

Attitude
The product of an individual's beliefs in the outcomes of the health behaviour in question and their evaluation of these outcomes

Subjective norms
The individual's beliefs about the value other people (individuals or groups) place on his or her health behaviour and the extent to which there is a motivation to follow these expectations

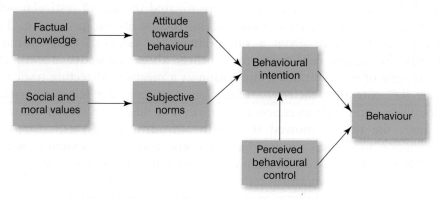

Figure 5.1 The theory of planned behaviour

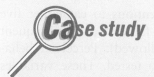

TPB – Chronic Illness

Alison is a physiotherapist who deals a lot with people who have chronic obstructive pulmonary disease (COPD) because she knows from her research that exercise can actually help people with COPD in terms of the severity of the condition if care is taken in designing an appropriate education campaign. Many patients feel that they cannot and should not exercise in case their condition gets worse and this is why she tries to help them, via physiotherapy.

Alan Jones is one of her patients she sees regularly. In a chat with him about appropriate exercise (for example chair based exercises) Alan tells her he thought that there was no point in exercising as his condition 'is going to get worse anyway' and that there is nothing he 'can do to stop it'. Alison corrects this misinformation informing him that mild exercise can help increase the function of his lungs, can help prevent chest infections (exacerbations)

and readmissions to hospital. He tells her that he loved exercising when he was younger particularly swimming. She informs him that with some clever use of his inhalers and good treatment there is no reason why he can't do some swimming again and that there is good evidence to say swimming really helps some people. He tells her that some of his friends say that you 'just have to take it easy' with this condition and Alison tells him that that is the case but it does not mean no exercise. She discusses his inhalers and some mild chair based exercises for now that he can do at home and leaves him to have a think about it before their next meeting in a couple of weeks' time.

Looking at the model of the Theory of Planned Behaviour can you identify:

1 Where Alan may be lacking in 'factual knowledge'?

2 Where his 'attitude towards exercise behaviour' may be important in helping Alison to assist him in changing his behaviour?

3 Where the 'subjective norms' of his friends may hinder his likelihood to change?

Brubaker and Wickersham (1990) investigated the use of testicular self-examination by young men following instruction in the procedure. The participants were also given a questionnaire to establish their attitudes towards this health behaviour, their beliefs about subjective norms, the effectiveness of testicular self-examination as a means of detecting testicular cancer (i.e. outcome), their own effectiveness at testicular self-examination (self-efficacy) and their intention to perform it in the future. When followed up later, the results showed that both attitude towards testicular self-examination and beliefs about subjective norms (such as the extent to which they felt other people wanted them to practise self-examination) significantly predicted intention to perform testicular self-examination.

Such findings suggest that screening rates might be improved by focusing on subjective norms – why other people might wish them to attend. In a similar vein, anti-smoking campaigns have featured a child looking beseechingly at a parent and saying 'But I don't want you to die!'

Povey *et al.* (2000) tested the TPB in the context of dieting. They used questionnaires to measure participants' initial intentions to eat either five portions of fruit and vegetables a day or a low-fat diet and subsequent behaviour (whether the dietary principle was followed). Perceived behavioural control, self-efficacy and beliefs were also tested. These variables were good predictors of intention to eat fruit and vegetables or reduce fat intake, with self-efficacy being a more consistent predictor than perceived control. In addition, attitude related strongly to intention to eat a low-fat diet and subjective norms predicted intention for eating fruit and vegetables. They concluded that self-efficacy was a better predictor of intention than perceived control, which suggests that a person's perception of their ability to engage in a behaviour is an important factor affecting their intention to perform that behaviour. So health promotion strategies that aim to change dietary habits should target people's attitudes and their self-efficacy.

Such findings have important implications for health promotion. Health behaviours that are strongly affected by the individual's attitudes are more likely to change if the individual is exposed to persuasive information but those behaviours that are primarily the product of subjective norms will be affected by attempts to change beliefs about expectations. Advice should also be specific and require an immediate change in behaviour.

Behaviours primarily driven by behavioural intention rather than perceived behavioural control also warrant a different approach to health promotion. Where behavioural intention is not the best predictor of behaviour, this raises the question, why not? The issue here is to ascertain the reasons why behaviour and intention are not related.

Stroebe (2000) suggests that such situations are rare and that, where behaviour is largely the product of perceived behavioural control, there is, in fact, very little variation in intention between individuals. Thus perceived behavioural control becomes a much more potent cause of action. More commonly, behaviour is governed predominantly by behavioural intention so, as well as the factors of attitude and subjective norms, the contribution of perceived behavioural control also has to be considered.

These findings have implications for improving health education. More emphasis should be given to changing attitudes, subjective norms and individuals' perception of their own effectiveness. However, it must be remembered that the TPB is predominantly intended to understand and predict intentions and behaviours rather than to provide a mechanism for behaviour change. So, like the HBM, the TPB may be able to identify the need for interventions, e.g. to change attitudes before behaviours, but it is quite difficult to develop interventions based on these variables, especially for the HBM. For example, Symons Downs and Hausenblas (2005) conducted a review of studies to explore the use of the TPB to understand exercise behaviour. They found key beliefs including that: exercise improves physical and psychological health, family members have the strongest normative influence on exercise, and that beliefs about physical limitations are the most in perceived behaviour control. So, whilst such findings indicate important areas of focus for behaviour change, such as targeting family members as well as the patient, or looking for strategies to overcome physical limitations, it may be difficult to find ways to implement these in practice. However, using a modified form of the TPB, Darker *et al.* (2010) devized an intervention intended to increase perceived behavioural control and found that this was effective in increasing walking in a sample of the general UK.

The transtheoretical model

Both the health belief model and the theory of planned behaviour (TPB) aim to identify factors that determine health behaviours and explain how they interact in order to predict whether or not an individual will perform a particular health behaviour. As these are both cognitive models, they only consider the variables involved in an individual's *thinking* about behaviour change, i.e. they assume that their decision is rational. However, our behaviour may also be non-rational – so may be difficult to bring under conscious control in order to achieve behaviour change. Other factors affecting behaviour change may be societal, for example differences in socioeconomic group or age or individual, such as the extent to which a person is wiling to change. Furthermore, because cognitive models focus on thinking, they do not consider the *type* of behaviour change needed. For instance, a patient with high blood pressure may need to *reduce* their salt intake, an obese person may need to develop a *new* habit of exercising, and a diabetic may need to *replace* some foods with different, and less appealing, ones. In order to achieve changes in health behaviours, it is important to discriminate between these requirements. These additional factors are considered in our final model, the transtheoretical model (TTM), Figure 5.2.

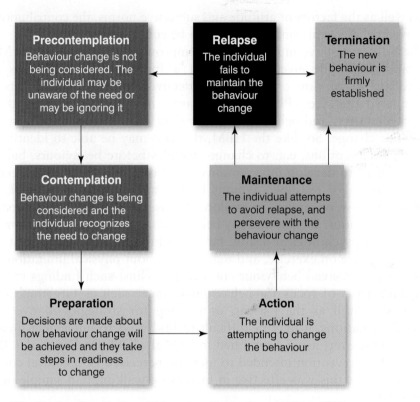

Figure 5.2   The transtheoretical model (based on *Prochaska and Velicer, 1997*)

The factors mentioned above contribute to an individual's readiness to change. This implies that changing behaviour is a process, something that a person 'works towards' over time rather than being a single event. This idea of progression is central to TTM, which suggests that behaviour change occurs systematically, and identifies stages distinguished by the individual's past behaviour and present intentions, so is also called the Stages of Change (SoC) theory. As it uses some of the same concepts as the cognitive models we have already discussed, it is called the *transtheoretical* model. Although the TTM suggests that the stages occur in order, an individual may regress, i.e. return to an earlier stage. One instance of this is 'relapse', in which a person who had changed their behaviour falls back into their previous habit. The model has been refined, so exists in several forms. The original, illustrated in the diagram below, has five stages, a more recent one has six (dividing 'action' into 'action planning' and 'implementation'). The five-stage version is more often referred to as it has been tested in more research. It offers a rough guide to the time an average person might spend in each stage, beginning with the precontemplation period when there is no foreseeable intention to change. Six months of contemplating the need to change is followed by a further month preparing for the change in behaviour. During the next 6 months the individual is engaged in action to make the change and post 6 months are deemed to be maintaining the behaviour. Maintenance continues until the behaviour is firmly established, after 5 to 6 years or more.

In addition to the stages, the model also incorporates ideas of:

- **Processes of change**: the covert and overt activities individuals use to progress through the stages. These are important because they offer health promotion opportunities (see Table 5.2).
- **Decisional balance**: a person's weighting of the relative importance of the costs and benefits of changing their behaviour. As individuals progress through the stages, the relative importance of benefits outweighs that of costs. This can indicate the specific help needed to assist progress.
- **self-efficacy** versus **temptation**: a person's situation-specific confidence in being able to avoid relapsing in a high-risk situation i.e. to resist temptation. This indicates potential ways to help the individual to stay on track.

The TTM is useful because it offers ways to measure an individual's progress, i.e. the extent to which their intentions and behaviour have changed and how stable these changes are likely to be. Another advantage of this model is the guidance it provides for promoting health (see Table 5.2). It allows health and social care professionals to see how they can tailor advice to specific needs. For example, counterconditioning and stimulus control are helpful for individuals in the action or maintenance stages but would be ineffective for those in precontemplation. Here, consciousness raising and dramatic relief are more used. The effectiveness of such tailoring of programmes was illustrated by Noar *et al.* (2007). In a **meta-analysis** of 57 studies, they found that health change interventions tailored according to the TTM were more effective than interventions that were not. Specifically, targeting by stage, on specific pros and cons (with regard to decisional balance), and on self-efficacy, produced better outcomes. Furthermore, TTM provides a way to find the best time to implement health promotion programmes. For example, Ohlendorf (2012) studied the stage of change of postpartum women with regard to their readiness to engage in weight self-management. Nearly half of the sample was in the contemplation stage during their postpartum hospitalization. This is therefore an ideal time for interventions to facilitate self-management of weight.

Haakstad *et al.* (2012) investigated the SoC of pregnant women with regard to engaging in physical activity. Over half of the women took regular exercise (i.e. were in the action or maintenance stages, 4 and 5) but very few had recently begun an exercise programme (entered stage 4). A third were doing only irregular physical activity. Those who had received advice from health and social care professionals were more likely to be in stages 4 or 5, and those for whom the decisional balance was weighted against exercising (e.g. pregravid overweight women or those with pelvic girdle pain) had low readiness to change exercise habits (stages 1–3). Importantly, pregnancy may offer an opportunity to make long-term changes to physical activity habits.

Meta-analysis
A statistical technique that combines the results of many studies

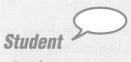

Student

Student nurse

Recognizing readiness for change

My mentor and I were dealing with a man who had been admitted to A&E many times with drinking related injuries. She talked to him about his drinking and it was clear that he had no intention of giving up his alcohol at all. To my surprise, my mentor started to speak to him about cutting down on drinking, drinking alcohol of a lesser strength and restricting his total intake. When I asked her about this she said the man was in precontemplation and that the best we could hope for was for him to reduce the harm to himself. I could understand this and that he was not ready to change.

Table 5.2	Processes of change	
Name of process	**Outline of process**	**Example of application**
Consciousness raising	*Increasing awareness*, e.g. taking notice of comments about the problem from friends, food labels on packets or information on the Internet	Information and education can be provided by health and social carers and personal feedback can be given about the healthy behaviour
Dramatic relief	*Emotional arousal* in response to increased awareness, e.g. reacting anxiously to warnings about smoking cigarettes	Providing inspirational examples of individuals who have changed their behaviour, giving the individual hope about their own capacity for lifestyle change
Environmental re-evaluation	*Social reappraisal*, e.g. considering the view that smoking is damaging to social and physical environment for themselves and other people	Illustrating how the individual's unhealthy behaviour is negatively affecting others and showing how this could be changed to produce positive effects
Self re-evaluation	*Self reappraisal* e.g. recognizing that one's inability to lose weight is disappointing	Helping patients to accept that healthy behaviour is an important part of their sense of who they are and who they want to be
Self liberation	*Committing* i.e. accepting one's determination to change and believing in one's capacity to do so	Facilitating the patient's self-belief, enabling them to make and stick to their commitments
Social liberation	*Environmental opportunities* e.g. realizing that society is changing in ways that make healthy behaviours easier	Helping the individual to recognize that society is more supportive of the healthy behaviour
Helping relationship	*Support* e.g. having somebody who will listen when the individual needs to talk about the health behaviour in question	Offering a listening ear, or identifying people who will be supportive of the behaviour change, including its difficulties
Stimulus control	*Re-engineering,* i.e. changing the immediate situation in order to make behaviour change easier	Giving advice or assistance to remove things from the social or physical surroundings, e.g. activities or the home, that trigger the behaviour to be changed

(Continued)

Table 5.2 Processes of change *(Continued)*		
Name of process	**Outline of process**	**Example of application**
Counter conditioning	*Substituting,* i.e. engaging better behaviours which can be substituted for unhealthy ones	Suggesting healthy ways of acting and thinking as alternatives for unhealthy ones
Reinforcement management	*Rewarding,* i.e. giving oneself a 'pat on the back' or a treat for doing the right thing or avoiding the wrong thing	Identifying suitable rewards to increase the frequency of healthy behaviours and helping individuals to reduce any good consequences of unhealthy behaviours

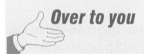

Over to you

Let's look at an example of how the TTM might work in practice. Imagine a counselling therapist faced with helping a client who has been advised to quit smoking. Initially they may feel that there is little point in trying as they are ill anyway, or that they know lots of perfectly healthy people who smoke, so what's all the fuss about. At this point the client is in the precontemplation stage. As they notice more symptoms, or recognize the reality of the dangers, they enter the contemplation stage and begin to think about giving up (the contemplation stage). This leads to investigating, or being amenable to advice about, strategies to help during the planning stage. The patient makes a decision about how to quit and tries to do so. Many factors will influence whether they succeed initially (maintenance) and whether this leads to them to abandon their efforts (relapse) or to become a non-smoker (termination).

Consider what the psychotherapist might do at each stage to assist the individual.

If the TTM model is to be helpful, it should be possible to track progress in behaviour change and to show that individuals who reach higher stages are more likely to take steps towards behaviour change and to ultimately achieve termination. This is generally the case, for example, Manne *et al.* (2002) found that people in higher stages of change were more likely to engage in testing for colorectal cancer and the same pattern was found by Lauver *et al.* (2003) for engagement in breast cancer screening.

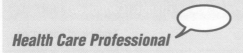

Health Care Professional

Physiotherapist

'It's really important for people to engage in physiotherapy post-operatively or after an injury but it can be really hard to motivate them to fully participate. For some, this relates to the fact that it can be painful and it's hard for them to believe that something which causes pain may be necessary although effective pain relief can make a significant difference. Others feel that an injured limb or back should be rested or immobilized because this is part of their cultural or family belief system. It can be hard to change someone's mind when they believe something strongly even if modern research supports the opposite. Clear communication and lots of encouragement can make a real difference.'

Key concepts

Motivational interviewing: This technique is based on cognitive behaviour therapy and uses one-to-one contact between the patient and a health and social care professional such as a counsellor or dietician. The aim is to enhance the client's determination to change by helping them to understand their own thoughts about the problem and how these lead to unhealthy behaviours so that they can see how they need to change in order to develop alternative, healthy habits. Techniques such as open-ended questions, reflecting and summarizing allow the patient to express their concerns and for these to be reinforced, showing how they are right to pay attention to the issue and possible courses of action, making it clear that the individual has choices. Questions can also be used to raise the individual's self-confidence, such as asking them what things they could do to help make the change, and asking them to rate their confidence and what they might do to make themselves more certain about managing to make the change. Successes can be built upon and failures can reframed, so they are less discouraging. For example, a client's comment that 'I've tried to diet so many times but just put it all back on' can be reframed as 'You have had several attempts at weight loss which have succeeded, you know you can lose the weight, so you already have strategies to help you start'. This can then lead to prompts to identify the need for new strategies, such as 'what do you think are the obstacles that prevent you from keeping the weight off?'

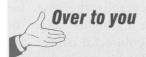

Over to you

Think about the kinds of questions and comments a motivational interviewer might ask and make in conversation with someone trying to quit smoking (consider open-ended questions, reflecting, summarizing, reinforcing concerns (affirmation), emphasizing choices, reframing, measuring and raising self-confidence, reviewing successes and eliciting coping strategies).

In addition, health and social care professionals using techniques based on the TTM should find that patients change their behaviour more readily. This, too, appears to be so. van Nes and Sawatzky (2010) found that health and social care professionals counselling cardiovascular patients see better outcomes with clients who are resistant and ambivalent to change with motivational interviewing than with traditional advice-giving. Jackson *et al.* (2007) found a similar pattern of success using a TTM-based strategy for behaviour change in diabetic patients (see Research in brief), which showed that it was more likely to lead to progression through the stages.

RESEARCH IN BRIEF

Jackson *et al.* (2007) Using the transtheoretical model to promote physical activity in people with diabetes.

Aim: To use the TTM to guide a behaviour change programme intended to increase physical activity in people with type 2 diabetes.

Procedure: Forty diabetic patients participated in either an experimental or a control group. All were given a physical activity leaflet. The experimental group also had an exercise consultation interview (ECI) designed to motivate physical activity. Physical activity levels and stage of change (SoC) were measured at the start of the programme and after 6 weeks.

Results: Physical activity levels increased in both groups but much more so in the ECI group, in which eight participants (almost half the group) increased their SoC whereas only one patient did so in the control group.

Conclusion: A TTM-based intervention is more likely to result in an increase in physical activity in people with diabetes than the standard provision of a leaflet.

Although studies have demonstrated the effectiveness of the TTM to direct the type and timing of health interventions, not all evidence supports the model. Cahill *et al.* (2010) conducted a review of many studies that looked, in various ways, at comparisons between smoking cessation programmes that were or were not tailored to the individual's stage. Although they found that stage-based interventions were effective, they were no more so than similar non-tailored interventions in terms of the likelihood of abstinence six months on from the start of treatment.

CHANGING HEALTH BEHAVIOURS THROUGH HEALTH EDUCATION PROGRAMMES

Health education programmes attempt to change people's health behaviours from health-compromising to health-enhancing ones. They may use different routes according to the model being followed. For example, fear-arousing appeals should, according to the health belief model, increase perceived vulnerability – but this approach has little success. Warner (1977) found only small, transient reductions in smoking (4–5 per cent) following scares in the USA in the 1950s and 1960s. It could also be argued that a 'shock–horror' approach to discouraging drug use is counter-productive for example by emphasizing the seductive qualities of a drug or by encouraging people to simply ignore the whole issue.

Informational appeals aim to promote health by providing people with the knowledge to make better health behaviour choices. However, information presented in campaigns may be interpreted differently by recipients from the way that was intended. In population terms, nearly 10 000 in every 1 000 000 male smokers aged 35 will die before reaching 45 because of their habit. From the perspective of the individual, however, this is only a 1 per cent chance – the odds are on survival. It is difficult to persuade individuals of the risk, so campaigns need to identify and focus on other routes to changing behaviour.

Nevertheless, access to information may still be a barrier. In presenting information to people in order to promote change, Taylor (1995) suggested that it should:

- be colourful, vivid, virtually statistics-free and use case histories
- come from an expert source
- discuss both sides of the issue
- have the strongest arguments at the beginning and end of the message
- be short and clear
- have explicit rather than implicit conclusions
- not be too extreme.

Reflective activity

Consider promotional material you have distributed to patients or have seen in hospitals or your local doctor's surgery. To what extent does it fulfil the criteria suggested by Taylor (1995)?

Raising awareness

As we have seen in relation to each of the theories, a key step in encouraging improved health behaviour is to increase awareness of healthy and unhealthy options.

Over to you

Major campaigns have been launched to raise awareness of specific risks, such as HIV infection and meningitis.

Look for resources relating to a recent campaign and consider the following questions. What kinds of messages are used to inform people? Do they impart knowledge? If so, does it relate to seriousness, vulnerability or other aspects of the disease? Does the information attempt to alter beliefs or attitudes? Do they try to influence subjective norms or people's perceptions, or their own behavioural control? Are the messages directed towards people who are not contemplating change, those considering it or those engaged in changing?

The three models of health behaviour we have considered, the health belief model, the theory of planned behaviour and the transtheoretical model all suggest that awareness is important in promoting health behaviours. The HBM suggests that awareness is essential to making assessments of vulnerability and seriousness that combine to enable the individual to judge the threat posed by a disease. In addition, knowledge about the benefits of a particular health behaviour and ways to overcome barriers enable the individual to sway their cost–benefit analysis in favour of engaging in healthier behaviours.

Awareness is also important from the perspective of the TPB. Here, knowledge is a prerequisite in the formation of attitudes towards health behaviours. Inadequate awareness or misinformation would lead to poor health behaviour choices; therefore it is the role of health promotion to ensure that people are aware of sufficient and appropriate resources so that they can make informed choices.

Finally, an acknowledgement that there is a problem to be solved is the key awareness that separates the precontemplation and contemplation stages in the TTM.

Over to you

Return to the following descriptions of studies reported earlier in this chapter:

- Horne *et al.* 2010 (p. 101)
- Manne *et al.* 2002 (p. 119)
- Lauver *et al.* 2003 (p. 119)
- Harvey and Lawson 2009 (p. 112)
- Darker *et al.* 2010 (p. 115)

For each study, identify the nature of the information that the participants needed in order to improve their awareness of health risks and justify your explanation using the HBM, the TPB or the TTM.

Persuasive communication and changing attitudes

As the models show, changing behaviours is not simply dependent on increasing knowledge – effective health promotion must change beliefs or attitudes for behaviour change to occur. For example, Kirscht *et al.* (1978) found that threat messages about weight control in obese children (which should have induced a change in maternal attitude) did indeed affect behaviour (the children lost weight). This shows that attitudes can affect behaviour. However, Leventhal and Cleary (1980) failed to change health behaviour; even when smokers' attitudes were manipulated by stimulating feelings of vulnerability they did not stop smoking. Similarly, despite their coverage, early television campaigns to reduce alcohol and drug abuse were unsuccessful (Morrison *et al.* 1976). Hovland (based at Yale University) developed a theory of persuasive communication in the 1950s (the 'Yale model') that laid the foundation for modern theories of attitude change, Figure 5.3.

In order for a communication to be persuasive it must first be noticed, thus attention is the first stage of the model. Individuals are unlikely to be influenced by 'Stop smoking' messages unless they are prominent. However, attending to the information alone does not guarantee attitude change, the recipient must also be able to understand the content. Comprehension is needed for persuasion to be successful. For example, if a hospital wants staff to follow a complex policy of segregating waste, but this is not clearly explained, they are unlikely to follow the procedure.

Whilst both attention and comprehension are necessary, they are not sufficient. Finally the message must be accepted. Acceptance does not necessarily demand belief but it does require that the receiver acts on their understanding. Thus, if we see a notice that says 'closing doors saves lives', we may not believe that our actions will be that significant but, because we understand the sentiment of the message, our behaviours change accordingly.

This notion of a staged sequence in the processing of persuasive information, referred to as systematic processing, requires the receiver to *think* about the message rather than just being a passive recipient. To account for some of the observed effects of persuasive communication, McGuire (1968) separated 'acceptance' into two stages, yielding and retention, and introduced a final stage, action. This version of the model differentiates

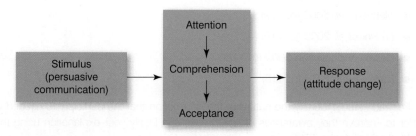

Figure 5.3   The Yale model of persuasive communication

between being persuaded by the message (yielding) and retaining that changed belief (retention). Patients with hypertension may see posters that advise them to cut down on salt and, although they understand and accept the message, they may forget why it was important. Thus, initially behaviour changes, i.e. there is action, but this may revert to inaction when retention fails. Incidentally, this staged progression refers to steps in the way we deal with information, rather than the stages of 'readiness to change' described by the TTM. However, the two are related in a sense – an individual in precontemplation does not progress beyond fleeting attention, an individual in contemplation attends and comprehends information but does not accept it. By the preparation stage the individual is making a response to the information they have received.

Factors affecting persuasion

In addition to describing the process of behaviour change, the Yale model indicates factors that influence the acceptance of persuasive communications. These factors are:

- The communicator of the message – the role, affiliations and intentions of the source.
- The content of the message – the topics, appeals, arguments and stylistic features.
- The media characteristics of the message – whether interaction is direct or indirect and the sensory modality used.
- The situational surroundings – such as the social setting and extraneous pleasant or unpleasant stimuli.
- The characteristics of the recipient – such as persuadability and self-confidence.

Communicator factors

The source of the message is an important factor in the success of attitude change. Some key factors include:

- The credibility and expertise of the source – communicators who are believable and perceived to be knowledgeable in their field are more effective.
- Communicators who argue against their own best interests – a nutritionist who says it is OK to eat some saturated fat is more likely to be believed than a dairy farmer who says the same thing.
- Attractiveness of the communicator – physically attractive individuals are more effective.
- Perceived similarity of the communicator to the recipient – this is particularly so if the similarity is deemed to be relevant to the issue.
- Likeability of the source – we are more readily persuaded by an individual whom we find pleasant than one we do not.

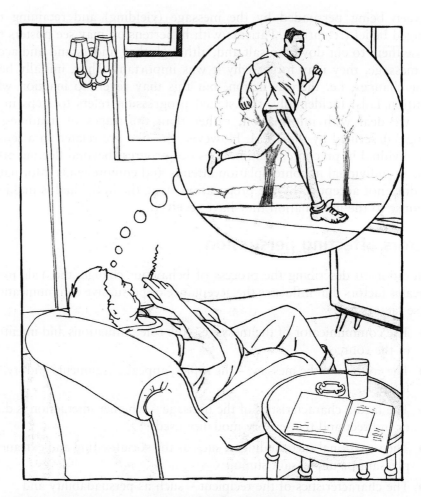

How would you motivate someone to get active and stop smoking?

Content factors

Many characteristics of the message are also important, these include:

- **Emotional content** – is it fear-arousing?
- **Medium** – verbal or visual?
- **Argument** – is it presented as a one-sided or two-sided debate?

A range of factors influence the effectiveness of fear-arousing arguments: the unpleasantness of the suggestion, the probability of the event occurring if the action is not followed; and the perceived effectiveness of the recommendation. Persuasive communication should therefore be most powerful if the recipient finds the suggestion relatively unpleasant, really believes it will happen and expects that the evasive action will be effective.

However, high levels of fear-arousal are not always the most effective. Janis and Feshbach (1953) found the reverse, with low levels of fear-arousal producing the most behaviour change. Thus, health messages about, for example, skin cancer and sunbathing that focus on avoiding wrinkles and getting sunburn may be more effective than threats about dying of cancer.

Some additional factors have been shown to affect attitude change. Howard (1997) demonstrated the power of familiarity. Students were more likely to be persuaded by an argument couched in familiar terms, such as 'Don't put all your eggs in one basket' or 'Don't bury your head in the sand', than one expressed in phrases such as 'Don't pretend a problem doesn't exist'. This links to the idea in the TPB that subjective norms – our beliefs about the opinions of others – matter to our potential for behaviour change.

Media factors

For messages geared towards encouraging healthy behaviour, which medium is most effective – or does it depend on the message being conveyed?

The answer seems to depend on when the recipient is likely to resist the message. If difficulties are likely to arise with comprehension, for instance if the message is complex, then written communications are most effective. If problems arise with yielding to the message, more direct media, such as face-to-face interactions, are better.

Thus, explaining the impact of high- and low-density lipoproteins on cholesterol level would be better presented on paper, since it is a relatively complex issue. In contrast, persuading schoolchildren to eat five portions of fruit or vegetables a day would be more successfully tackled face to face, as the problem is not one of difficulty with understanding but of encouraging participation.

Situational factors

Presenting a communication as either a one-sided or two-sided argument can be advantageous in different situations. Where views are likely to be unopposed, a one-sided argument will achieve opinion change more quickly, if only temporarily. However, in many health-related situations, one view is likely to be countered by another: non-smokers by smokers for example. In these instances, persuasive communication is more likely to be effective if both sides of the argument are acknowledged.

In these instances, primacy and recency effects come into play. If the time lag between the presentation of the two sides of the issue is small, the first message should be more effective (because of the primacy effect). If, however, the interval is long, the later message will be better remembered, because of the recency effect, so is likely to result in greater attitude change (Petty and Cacioppo, 1981).

So, in a debate about the merits of health and social care professionals undergoing basic care training, the first speaker is advantaged because the presentations are likely to follow one another in quick succession. However, if cases are to be presented in a monthly bulletin in successive editions, there is a distinct advantage in being the last to appear.

Reflective activity

A local community group is campaigning for the loan of medical equipment such as wheelchairs and transcutaneous electrical neurological stimulation (TENS) machines to be free but this is being opposed by health centre managers. If you represented either the local community or the health centre management and could design screen savers to appear on every local library computer monitor for 1 week, would you choose the first week or the second? If each group were allocated an afternoon to give presentations to the residents' association, would you rather speak first or last? If your message was complex, would you opt for the verbal presentation or a written message on the computers?

Another situational factor affecting the persuasiveness of communication is the nature of the distractions with which it has to compete. It seems obvious that a message will be less effective if it is in competition with other stimuli because distractions prevent rehearsal and therefore impair memory. However, this is not always the case. While a viewpoint with which an individual agrees may be disadvantaged by interruptions (they are less able to focus on the additional supporting arguments), a contrary viewpoint may benefit from distractions. If an individual is attending to a message that conflicts with their prevailing view, but is distracted, they will be unable to generate their own arguments against it; thus it will seem more persuasive.

Social skills training

Relaxation therapy
A therapeutic approach applied to many different contexts, which aims to reduce tension and produce a state of calmness and can use several different techniques. One common one is to focus on breathing slowly and progressively contracting and relaxing muscles blocks.

Social skills training can be used to enable people to identify their personal and social needs and to develop the skills required to meet their health needs. For instance, many smokers report that they smoke to reduce social anxiety, so finding alternative means to relax could be beneficial. Since the largest group of new smokers is young people, they need to gain the necessary social skills to avoid taking up smoking at all. This can be achieved with **relaxation therapy**, allowing individuals alternatives to smoking for coping with difficult situations. Self-management strategies used with smokers encourage the participant to monitor the circumstances under which smoking occurs. Self-reward techniques can then be used to separate smoking behaviour from the environmental cues with which it is associated.

RESEARCH IN BRIEF

Steptoe *et al.* (1999) Confidence of practice nurses in conveying cardiovascular health advice.

Aim: To assess perceptions and effectiveness of nurses and GPs with regard to giving lifestyle counselling to cardiovascular patients.

Procedure: A questionnaire was given to 107 GPs and 58 practice nurses from 19 group practices. There was a 100 per cent response rate.

Results: Nurses were perceived to have the main responsibility for cardiovascular health promotion and attitudes to the role were generally positive. A lack of training in offering counselling was a problem and greater confidence in training was linked to confidence in effectiveness and a positive attitude to health promotion. However, few responders believed they were very effective in changing lifestyles: variously, cigarette smoking, physical inactivity and obesity were seen as difficult to change. There was no link between the respondents' own health behaviours and their attitudes to health promotion.

Conclusion: Staff recognize that health promotion is more than just the provision of information and advice but are not confident that they have the skills to implement prevention strategies effectively.

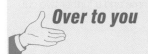 **Over to you**

Using any of the health models, suggest ways that social skills training might be important.

Johnson *et al.* (2008) conducted a review of studies of behavioural interventions to reduce HIV infection in men who sleep with men (MSM). Using the findings of 44 studies, evaluating 58 interventions with 18 585 participants, they identified several key patterns and developed many useful suggestions for research. For example, they found that interventions were more effective for non-gay identified MSM, probably because they would have had less previous exposure to prevention. For this group, training in skills such as keeping condoms available and behavioral self-management is worthwhile.

RESEARCH IN BRIEF

Whittaker *et al.* (2008) A multimedia mobile phone-based intervention smoking cessation programme for young people.

Aim: To develop a video and text-message based intervention to reduce smoking in young people.

Procedure: A selection of multimedia resources was developed in consultation with young people, who recognized the need for, amongst other things, relevant role models and music for relaxation. A young student who had recently quit smoking herself was selected to record her experiences in a chronological series of messages. Each one was based on an issue associated with how the model coped, giving messages on how to keep motivated and stay quit, such as dealing with stress and goal setting. The use of phone technology and varied, high-quality multimedia material helped to encourage the participants to persevere, as did the availability of the messages which were sent automatically and could be received anywhere, anytime. In addition to the automatic messages, participants could request extra support on demand to receive immediate tips on managing cravings. Video clips were also included produced by high school students about the proven ill effects of smoking. The whole chronological sequence started with the lead-up to Quit Day, Quit Day messages and then post–Quit Day.

The participants themselves were 13 young people, aged 16 years or older and were daily smokers who wanted to quit. Over a 4-week period, all the role model quit diary interspersed with the anti-tobacco videos and text messages. At the end they were telephoned to complete a telephone questionnaire.

Results: Nine participants stopped smoking during the programme and a further two cut down. Those who quit felt that the programme had helped.

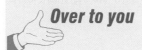

Over to you

The study described above incorporates many ideas from each of the models we have discussed as well as illustrating many of the other points raised in the chapter. Write a list extracting as many ideas from the study as you can, identifying how each can be justified.

CONCLUSIONS

Primary prevention strategies aim to encourage positive health behaviours by providing information that warns of risks to health without inducing fear. Such strategies can improve health behaviours. In the case of healthy eating, biological explanations suggest that genetic factors, such as the predisposition to obesity, affect our health. Metabolic rate, fat cells and weight all have inherited components. Eating habits may also be acquired, by classical or operant conditioning and through social learning. Foods may become associated with emotional states and may act as a reinforcer (or punisher). We may imitate the amount or types of food that role models consume. Cultural factors may also determine health behaviours such as the types of food we eat and when we eat them.

The health belief model explains health behaviours by considering how we process information about health. It suggests that, in relation to any health behaviour, we have five central beliefs about our vulnerability, the seriousness of the condition, potential barriers to and benefits of taking evasive action and cues that trigger the behaviour. When these variables favour action over inaction, positive health behaviour should occur. This explanation can successfully account for preventative behaviours such as immunizations and self-examination and for attendance or non-attendance at screening tests.

The theory of planned behaviour suggests that health behaviours are determined by the intention to act and the extent of perceived behavioural control. When an individual both intends to engage in a health behaviour and feels that they have the power to do so, they will take action. Intention is determined by knowledge, attitudes and subjective norms while perceived behavioural control is affected by self-efficacy as well as intrinsic motivation and external factors. The theory can help to direct health campaigns by identifying why people fail to engage in health behaviours.

The transtheoretical model goes further than the other two models, describing the stages an individual passes through as they decide to change their behaviour, and implement that change, as well as the factors involved – the processes of change. The model therefore clearly indicates for when and how behaviour change happens, potentially tailoring strategies to individuals' needs. This has been particularly effective in targeting interventions for smoking cessation and for healthy eating.

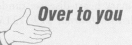

Over to you

Consider how you would develop and test your own health education strategy, based on one of the models. Once you have decided on the model and a health behaviour to promote, it may help to draw out a large copy of the model, inserting the factors that you think are relevant to the issue you are exploring.

RAPID RECAP

Check your progress so far by working through each of the following questions.

1 What influences behaviour change according to the health belief model?

2 What are the key elements in the theory of planned behaviour?

3 How does an individual progress through the stages of change according to the transtheoretical model and what role do the processes of change play in their progress?

4 The following factors could affect an individual who is thinking about giving up smoking: the existence of many non-smoking restaurants; the belief that smoky clothes is unpleasant; a desire to combat the effects of smoking on their asthma; the knowledge that they can stop themselves from starting again once they have said they've given up. Explain how these factors would relate to each of the models.

5 Use one model to suggest several ways to help a group of obese children to improve their eating habits.

If you have difficulty with any of the questions, read through the section again to refresh your understanding before moving on.

KEY REFERENCES

Other references are listed on the supporting website.

Blake, Malik, Phoenix and Pisano (2011) 'Do as I say, but not as I do': Are next generation nurses role models for health? *Perspectives in Public Health* 131 (5) 231–239.

Horne, P.J., Greenhalgh, J., Erjavac, M., Lowe, C.F., Viktor, S. and Whitaker, C.J. (2011) Increasing pre-school childrens consumption of fruit and vegetables. A modelling and rewards intervention. *Appetite.* 56 (2) 375–385.

Jackson, R., Asimakopoulou, K. and Scammell, A. (2007) Assessment of the transtheoretical model as used by dietitians in promoting physical activity in people with type 2 diabetes. *Journal of Human Nutrition and Diet* 20 (1) 27–36.

Janis, I.L. and Feshbach, S. (1953) Effects of fear-arousing communications. *Journal of Abnormal and Social Psychology*, **48**: 78–92.

Steptoe, A., Doherty, S., Rink, E., Kerry, S., Kendrick, T. and Hilton, S. (1999) Behavioural counselling in general practice for the promotion of healthy behaviour among adults at increased risk of coronary heart disease: randomised trial. *British Medical Journal* 319 (7215): 943–947.

Whittaker, R., Maddison, R., McRobbie, H., Bullen, C., Denny, S., Dorey, E., Ellis-Pegler, M., van Rooyen, J. and Rodgers, A. (2008) *Journal of Medical Internet Research* 10 (5) e49.

CHAPTER 6

ADHERENCE TO TREATMENT

LEARNING OBJECTIVES

By the end of this chapter you should be able to:

- explain what is meant by patient non-adherence

- describe and evaluate methods for assessing adherence

- explain patient-related factors that help to understand why patients may not follow instructions given to them by health and social care professionals

- explain practitioner-related factors that help to understand why patients may not follow instructions given to them by health and social care professionals

- identify and justify good practice that would help patients to understand, remember and act on advice.

P atients receiving treatment from their health and social care providers are exposed to information. This can vary from relatively simple details about when and how to take medicine prescribed by the GP to complex anatomical information, relating to a serious illness and possible treatment options. The patients must comprehend and remember this information and then act on it. The advice they are given for action may include not just drug regimes but instructions on diet, abstaining from or reducing smoking or alcohol consumption, taking rest or exercise, avoiding stress and attending future appointments. In many cases, patients do not follow these instructions. In this chapter we explore the reasons why patients may fail to follow medical advice and look at how this problem may be reduced.

IS NON-ADHERENCE A PROBLEM?

Early research in this area referred to compliance with medical advice, implying that non-compliant patients were being deliberately 'disobedient' when they failed to follow instructions. This is now being replaced with the term *adherence*, suggesting that the patient may, or may not, 'stick to' the advice given. This is preferable as it recognizes that:

- Patients have choices and may be opting not to follow instructions.
- When patients do not follow advice, the reason may be because they cannot rather than they will not.
- Patient–practitioner communication is a co-operative process rather than a one-way channel.

Many patients do not adhere to the advice they are given, although estimates of non-adherence rates vary with patient group, research method and definition of adherence. Ley and Llewelyn (1995) provide a comparison of reported non-adherence rates in different medical settings and for a range of types of advice obtained from different research sources. The results demonstrate a considerable problem, with non-adherence being consistently high, ranging from 39.5 per cent to 60 per cent. Such findings suggest that patients are not benefiting as much as they could from the information and follow-up care provided for them by health and social care professionals.

Reflective activity

Have you ever not adhered to a medical treatment? If so, why did you not complete it or even start it? Ask some friends and family the same question. Are there any similarities?

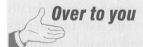 **Over to you**

You have been asked to measure how well people stick to a drug and exercise treatment for hypertension. Explain how you would measure successful adherence. Justify your answer.

KEY POINTS

- Non-adherence by patients is common, with perhaps more than 50 per cent of patients not following advice given.
- Non-adherence may be rational and deliberate, or unintentional.
- Health and social care professionals also demonstrate non-adherence in relation to work guidelines and regulations.

PREDICTING AND EXPLAINING ADHERENCE AND NON-ADHERENCE

There are several possible reasons why patients may not follow medical advice that they have been given. These include:

- Not being aware of the information (e.g. if they have not listened to advice or looked at a leaflet).
- Being unable to understand the advice, so unable to follow it.
- Not believing advice to be true, or to be relevant to themselves.
- Not being able to recall the information in order to follow it.
- Not having the motivation to persist with following advice.
- Being unable to cope with the requirements of following the advice.
- Choosing to ignore advice or to follow a different course of action.

There are several theories that can help us to understand the causes of adherence and how it may be increased. In this chapter we will consider a behavioural and a cognitive model of compliance, two models of memory, the parallel response model and also the two models of health behaviour discussed in Chapter 5. Each of these helps us to understand a different aspect of adherence.

THE BEHAVIOURAL MODEL OF COMPLIANCE

One explanation for the acquisition and performance of behaviours is operant conditioning. This theory of learning forms the basis for the behavioural model of compliance. The major proponent of operant conditioning, B.F. Skinner, identified several key mechanisms that determine whether behaviours are repeated. He suggested that an individual (human or animal) performs a random variety of behaviours and, of those, some are reinforced (result in pleasant consequences that increase the frequency of the behaviour) while others are punished (result in unpleasant consequences that decrease the frequency of the behaviour). These behaviours may be responses to certain stimuli or cues in the environment.

Reinforcement in the context of adherence to medical advice includes health benefits such as reduction in pain or other unpleasant symptoms (this type of reinforcement, in which good consequences derive from the removal of something unpleasant, is called negative reinforcement). An example of negative reinforcement can be seen in the relief a patient feels when their health improves and they no longer feel a burden to others – the removal of that pressure feels good so acts as a reinforcer to promote further improvement. Other reinforcers could include praise from a health practitioner, feeling more energetic or losing weight. As these are good experiences, they are examples of positive reinforcement.

A technique called shaping, also based on operant conditioning, can be used to modify behaviours. This employs positive reinforcement to reward behaviours that more closely resemble the desired outcome. For example, patients with hypertension could be rewarded for progressively excluding unsuitable foods from their diet. Initially they would be reinforced for making straightforward adjustments to their diet, such as changes to LoSalt, then subsequently for making more difficult refinements to their intake, such as altering the way that they cook individual meals.

Punishment is less effective than reinforcement as a way to change behaviour, in part because it offers no alternative behaviour, it simply aims to suppress the performance of an action. Punishments could include the fear induced by threats, such as telling children their teeth will rot if they don't brush them. The unpleasant effects of failure to adhere to advice, such as the threats to health caused by smoking, cannot act as effective punishers as they are not contingent – they do not immediately follow the performance of the behaviour.

The behavioural model would therefore predict that adherence would be best when there are appropriate and contingent reinforcers for performing the behaviours advised and, possibly, if non-adherent behaviour is punished. In reality, there may be many instances in which the reverse is true. Adherence itself may require commitments or lifestyle changes that are undesirable, such as extra time spent preparing a special diet, having to eat less palatable (but healthier) food, swallowing foul-tasting medicine or taking exercise. In addition, medication may have side-effects. These consequences, if perceived to be unpleasant, act as punishers so would tend to reduce the likelihood of compliance. Conversely, the potentially reinforcing benefits of adherence are unlikely to be immediate, or even short term. Therefore the consequences, even for good compliers, cannot act as positive reinforcers because their effects are not contingent upon the behaviours required by adherence. Indeed, for a patient for whom the sick role has become a way of life, recovery and therefore adherence, may represent a very frightening and powerful punisher.

The behavioural model has the advantage that the effects of reinforcers and punishers on behaviour can be seen and, as such, measured. Consequently, the effectiveness of behavioural interventions is relatively easy to identify. However, the behavioural model gives us no insight into the thought processes that underlie adherent or non-adherent behaviour.

THE COGNITIVE MODEL OF COMPLIANCE

Ley (1981) and Ley and Llewelyn (1995) have proposed a model, Figure 6.1, that considers the patient's thinking and attempts to predict whether patients will comply with medical advice. It suggests that compliance or non-compliance is determined by three factors:

- understanding
- memory
- satisfaction.

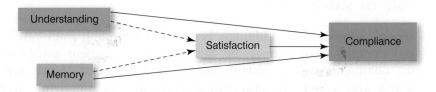

Figure 6.1 Ley's cognitive model of compliance

This is a cognitive model because it suggests that the determinants of compliance are processes related to thinking. According to the model, all three factors can affect compliance directly; better understanding, memory and greater satisfaction can each lead to a greater likelihood of compliance. In addition, the model suggests that patients who understand and remember the information that their health and social care professional has supplied are more likely to be satisfied and, as an indirect consequence, are more likely to comply. These stages have been explored through research that we will consider in the following sections.

The role of understanding

Kerr *et al.* (2003) found that 39 per cent of rectal cancer patients reported that there were aspects of communication with their clinician that were either incomprehensible or insufficient. This was particularly problematic for younger patients and those in larger hospitals. Armstrong *et al.* (1990) found little agreement between doctors and patients about whether or not a subsequent appointment had been recommended.

Patients who understand the information they are required to follow are more likely to adhere to it. For example, Ley *et al.* (1975) conducted an experiment to compare medication errors made by psychiatric patients using printed information that differed in difficulty. Those patients given leaflets with easier words and shorter sentences made fewer errors. Jones *et al.* (2012) noted that a lack of understanding via lower literacy levels affected adherence to treatment and testing for HIV and AIDS. People who fell into this category were much more likely to miss appointments and not know how their illness was progressing presumably as they had difficulty in comprehending how the disease is treated. Evidence such as this suggests that a significant proportion of patients may not understand instructions and, as a consequence, cannot comply.

The relationship between understanding and compliance is not, however, always a simple one. Hamburg and Inoff (1982) studied adolescents with diabetes who were attending a summer camp and found an inverted U relationship – that is, adherence was worst for individuals with very poor or very good understanding of their condition and its treatment. It is possible that individuals with an intermediate level of knowledge are the best compliers because they have sufficient understanding to follow the advice but, because they are unaware of the long-term implications, they are less afraid so are not discouraged.

The role of satisfaction

Ley's model suggests that, although better understanding does result in improved compliance, this may be due in part to patient satisfaction. Recently, Bhattacharya *et al.* (2012) discovered that around 25 per cent of their sample who were taking oral chemotherapy did not adhere fully to the treatment. Whilst satisfaction for things like the duration of therapy and how to know if the drug was working was around 60 per cent, the 40 per cent who were dissatisfied were not always the ones who did not adhere! Therefore, it might not be a clear-cut relationship between satisfaction and adherence – people may feel unsatisfied but they still take their medicine.

However, Dang *et al.* (2013) examined the role of satisfaction in adherence to HIV treatment in Texas. Patients were asked about their satisfaction with current treatment and their visits to the health clinics treating them. Patient satisfaction was directly linked to retention at the clinics, which in turn affected the likelihood that they would continue with the antiviral therapy. Patient satisfaction also directly affected the continuation of antiviral therapy irrespective of clinic visits. Therefore, patient satisfaction had a powerful effect on the adherence to treatment in this sample. This may show us that satisfaction could affect different diseases in different ways.

The role of cognitive factors

One reason why patients may fail to adhere to medical advice is that they cannot remember it. For example, Kravitz *et al.* (1993) found that, although 90 per cent of patients with a chronic condition could recall advice about medication, fewer remembered guidance about changes to their diet or exercise habits. Of those who did recall the advice, adherence ranged from 20 per cent for adherence to recommendations about exercise to 90 per cent for adherence to advice on medication.

In the following sections we will explore psychological explanations of memory and forgetting that can help us to understand why patients may forget what they are told. There have been many investigations studying patients' recall of medical information. These have used a range of techniques and sampled different groups of people. Such differences in approach have led to widely differing estimates of recall. Ley (1988) reviewed many such studies and found an overall average recall of around 50 per cent with estimates from different sources ranging from 28 per cent to 88 per cent. Clearly a lot of patients forget a great deal of what has been communicated to them. Why is this?

Some factors seem to reliably affect recall. Some key influences include:

- **Anxiety**: more anxious patients seem to have better recall.
- **Medical knowledge**: patients with greater knowledge have better recall.
- **Primacy effect**: patients have better recall for the first information presented to them.

- **Importance:** statements perceived by the patient to be important are recalled better.
- **Volume of information:** when more information is presented, more is recalled but the percentage remembered is lower (Broome and Llewelyn, 1995).

The influences on memory described above, and other effects on recall, can be explained by looking at two theories of memory; the multistore model and levels of processing theory.

Existing medical knowledge

In an experimental study, Brown and Park (2002) found that both younger and older participants learned more information about an unfamiliar disease than a familiar one. They concluded that health and social care professionals should consider that patients may have difficulty recalling new information about familiar diseases. This may be accounted for, at least in part, because new information about a condition may contradict existing knowledge. Rice and Okun (1994) found that medical information that conflicted with patients' existing beliefs was recalled less accurately than information that did not. Such findings are supported by psychological evidence relating to interference in memory.

Forgetting triggered by new information may be initiated in two ways. Proactive inhibition, as seen in these examples, arises when we have to learn new facts but old ones 'get in the way'. We experience this when we persist in writing last year's date on cheques well into February or answer the telephone in our new house with the old telephone number. In contrast, new memories can also 'overwrite' and obliterate old ones. When we learn a new PIN number or car registration, we experience difficulty recalling the previous one, a process called retroactive inhibition.

However, having knowledge about your own illness may be a positive thing with respect to adherence. Jones *et al.* (2012) noted that patients who had knowledge about their own HIV status were twice as likely to adhere to appointments compared to those who did not know their CD4 count or viral load. Knowledge about HIV appeared to be valuable in getting patients to continue treatment and control their symptoms and progression of the disease.

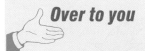

Over to you

Take one of the factors already discussed (e.g. role of understanding, role of satisfaction) and try to find some more studies that have tested it out. Pay particular attention to how they measured adherence and note what results the study found.

THE MULTISTORE MODEL OF MEMORY

The multistore model of memory, Figure 6.2, (Atkinson and Shiffrin 1968) suggests that incoming information is passed through three memory stores, each holding information for longer than the last. The first, the short-term sensory store (STSS), lasts only a matter of seconds, passing some but not all of its information on. If we fail to pay attention to information it will be lost at this stage. The remaining information is passed on the short-term memory (STM). This store last for about 30 seconds, although by repetition or rehearsal information can be kept in STM for longer. It is this same process of rehearsal that results in the transfer of information to the most permanent store, the long-term memory (LTM).

Rehearsal

If we do not have the opportunity to 'play the information over' in our minds, then new information will not be transferred from STM to LTM and will be forgotten. Patients may find that they need to ask health and social care professionals to repeat instructions or explanations in order to remember. Staff and patients may find this frustrating but rehearsal is one way to improve recall. MacKinnon and Fenaughty (1993) found that users of cigarettes, smokeless tobacco products and alcohol, who had therefore experienced greater exposure to health warnings had more opportunity to rehearse these messages, and hence demonstrated better recall for the content of such labels than non-users.

Displacement

Our short-term memory (STM) has a limited capacity. We can only store about seven items at a time; any more than this and new information starts to push older information out of STM before it has been transferred to LTM. This cause of forgetting is called **displacement**. If a health and social care professional answers a patient's question but then immediately follows this with a question themselves without giving the patient the opportunity to rehearse the information, the original answer may be displaced and forgotten.

Displacement
A cause of forgetting

So, if patients receive too many pieces of information at one time, they may begin to 'lose' some of the items. An item or 'chunk' is a single piece of

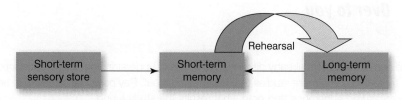

Figure 6.2   The multistore model of memory

information. To a patient, for whom medical information is novel, each fact will be a separate chunk occupying a space in STM. This makes the material harder to remember for patients than it is for experienced professionals.

The process of displacement can account for the primacy effect, the tendency to have better recall for the earliest items presented. Murdock (1962) conducted an experiment in which participants heard a list of words then had to recall words from different parts of the list. They were best at remembering items from the beginning (the primacy effect) and the end (called the recency effect). Their recall for items from the middle of the list was poor. The primacy effect arises because the early items are rehearsed and transferred from STM to LTM. Patients therefore have good recall for the earliest information they are given (Ley, 1972; 1982). Later items may be displaced by additional incoming information. More recently, Andrews and Carroll (1998) have also found a marked primacy effect in the memory for medical information.

It may be difficult for practitioners to see why patients have difficulty. As we saw in Chapter 2, health and social care practitioners have a 'register' or professional language which, when used inappropriately with less informed patients, is perceived as unintelligible jargon. Familiarity with words or ideas enables you to make bigger 'chunks'. When you first began to learn about psychology you probably had to spell the word letter by letter or in two 'sections' or chunks; now – hopefully – you can write the whole word without thinking. It has become a single chunk that takes up correspondingly less space in STM.

So, patients have two problems relating to displacement. First, information may be presented very quickly, so they don't have time to rehearse ideas and transfer them to LTM before they are displaced by later information. Second, because the concepts and terms are unfamiliar they cannot chunk the information so their STM fills up more quickly and displacement is more likely to occur.

KEY POINTS

- Information must be rehearsed in order to be transferred from STM to LTM, otherwise it will be forgotten.
- If more than approximately seven chunks of information are presented quickly, the early ones will be displaced and forgotten rather than transferred to LTM.

THE LEVELS OF PROCESSING THEORY OF MEMORY

Craik and Lockhart (1972) proposed the levels of processing theory of memory. This suggests that our memory consists of only one store but that information within it may be retained in different ways. According to Craik and Lockhart, by dealing with or 'processing' information more deeply, we are more likely to remember it. Deep or semantic processing occurs when we think about the meaning of information, for example, when we are trying to understand how an organ of the body works or why one course of treatment is better than another. There are three levels of processing:

> **Semantic processing**
> When we think about the meaning of information

- Structural processing relies only on superficial aspects, such as what an item looks like. For example, a patient may know the shape of the tablets they take or the colour of the box, or remember that following the red line through the hospital will get them to the X-ray department and the green line to the plaster room. It is the shallowest level of processing and results in the poorest recall.

- Phonemic processing uses information about the sound of the item to be remembered, for example if it sounds like another word or whether items rhyme. Children using preventer and reliever inhalers might remember 'use **br**own after **br**eakfast, keep **blue** with **you**'. It results in better recall than structural processing because it is deeper.

- Semantic processing deals with the meaning of information. It is the deepest level of processing and results in the best recall.

When patients are given information they need to be able to process it deeply in order to remember it but this may not be possible if they do not understand the concepts being discussed. Patients may be unfamiliar with bodily processes such as circulation so find the action of vasodilators or antihypertensives hard to comprehend. It is important therefore to ensure that patients receive sufficient explanation and that it is presented in an accessible way.

ILLNESS, TREATMENT AND ADHERENCE

Factors relating to the individual's condition, such as its severity, whether they are in pain and the nature of the treatment, are also important in explaining variability in adherence.

Seriousness of the illness and patient pain

It is a surprising finding that a patient who, according to their doctor, has a serious illness is no more likely to adhere to advice than one with a minor complaint. In fact, Haynes (1979) observed that 'not a single study has found that increasing severity of symptoms encourages compliance' (p. 51). A typical finding, from Vincent (1971), showed that more than half the glaucoma patients studied did not follow simple advice to use eye drops and even when their vision deteriorated to the extent that they were legally blind in one eye the compliance rate was still below 60 per cent. In contrast, both the severity of the illness, as perceived by the patient, and their experience of pain predicted adherence (Becker and Maiman, 1980; Becker, 1979).

The parallel response model

One explanation for these observations is offered by Leventhal's parallel response model (Leventhal, 1970). This suggests that, in a situation perceived to be dangerous, as could be the case with a serious illness, the individual appraises the threat in two independent ways:

- **Danger control**: motivation that results in adaptive behaviour to reduce the danger, such as following health advice, in order to overcome fear.
- **Fear control**: motivation directed towards reducing fear, such as ignoring symptoms and advice and engaging in maladaptive behaviours like drinking that may offer comfort in the short term.

If a patient is more highly motivated to control their fear than the danger, perhaps because they have little faith in the efficacy of treatment or are very afraid (as may arise in the case with diagnosis of a serious illness), Leventhal's model suggests that they are unlikely to adhere to advice. The model can therefore explain the lack of relationship between severity of illness and adherence.

When treatment is unpleasant: side-effects and time

Another surprising finding is that, contrary to logic, patients are as likely to be compliant when medication is unpleasant as when there are no side-effects (Masur, 1981). However, in some cases, side-effects could be sufficient to induce rational non-adherence. For example, Bulpitt *et al.* (1989) found that medication for hypertension that was successful in reducing symptoms such as headaches and depression also had side-effects resulting in sexual difficulties such as impotence. As we saw earlier, the behavioural model can account for non-adherence when undesirable side-effects act as punishers.

Patients are, however, less likely to comply when treatment is prolonged. Haynes (1976) found that compliance rates fell as treatment duration increased – patients are more likely to drop out from longer treatment programmes than shorter ones. This finding may alternatively be attributable to the nature of different conditions. Those requiring sustained attention, such as high blood pressure, may have fewer symptoms to trigger compliance. Patients may therefore fail to adhere to treatment in the absence of evidence of their own illness rather than because the duration of treatment is lengthy.

DiMatteo and DiNicola (1982) reported that, while 70–80 per cent of patients adhered to short-term medication regimens, less than 60 per cent stuck to preventative programmes and even fewer – not even 50 per cent – adhered to medical advice that required lifestyle changes. This illustrates another issue. Treatment for acute conditions, such as medication, requires little change to routine or habits so is relatively easy to adhere to. Following advice for the management of chronic conditions will more often require a significant lifestyle change, in diet, exercise or habits such as smoking. To consistently adhere to such recommendations demands a significantly greater effort on the part of the patient.

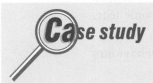

Martin and physiotherapy

Martin is a 30 year-old man who lives with his family in a council flat. For the last 10 years he has worked as a labourer in a building site and has developed chronic low back pain, which he feels is due to his job. Martin has been taking medication to relieve his pain and has also been seeing a physiotherapist recently on the recommendation of his doctor to help with his mobility. However, Martin finds the physiotherapy sessions uncomfortable and has started missing some appointments. When his physiotherapist asks him about this Martin tells her that he doesn't have time to do the exercises at home and feels that physiotherapy must be making his condition worse as it can hurt when he does the recommended movements. He believes that he should rest as much as possible to help his back and keep taking medication to get better. Martin's physiotherapist explains to him that the experience of pain during his exercises doesn't mean that the treatment is doing any damage to his body. She negotiates with Martin a revised treatment plan that he feels comfortable with and helps him to make a plan so that he can accommodate exercises in his life.

1 Why did the patient not adhere to his physiotherapy treatment?

2 What action did the physiotherapist take to empower the patient to engage with his treatment?

3 What additional strategies could be employed to maximize engagement with treatment?

The complexity of treatment

Cramer *et al.* (1989) found that as treatment becomes more complex (when more drug doses must be taken each day) adherence falls:

- One daily dose: 88 per cent adherence
- Three daily doses: 77 per cent adherence
- Four daily doses: 39 per cent adherence.

This pattern may arise because for one, two or three daily doses patients can identify an existing pattern to follow ('on waking', 'morning and night' or 'after meals'). This breaks down for a regime requiring four daily doses.

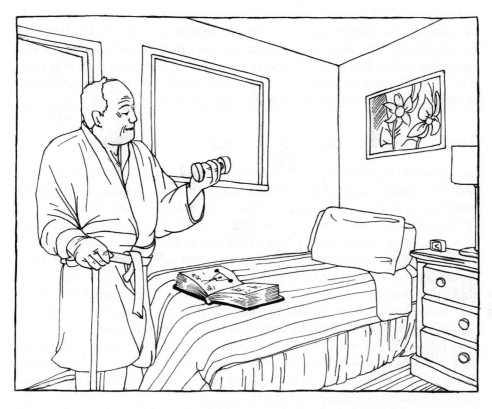

Why might this man give up doing the exercises given to him by his physiotherapist?

ADHERENCE AND CHARACTERISTICS OF THE INDIVIDUAL

Are some people more likely to comply than others? This section looks at a range of factors that affect the incidence of adherence in different individuals.

Reflective activity

Before reading on, think about patients you know that have not adhered to treatment. Why do you think they did not? See if any of your ideas feature in the next section!

Gender

In some respects, men and women are equally compliant, for example in taking medication for hypertension (Monane *et al.*, 1996). However, women are more likely to take medication for schizophrenia (Sellwood and Tarrier, 1994) and to follow dietary advice about the consumption of fruit and vegetables (Laforge *et al.*, 1994).

Holt *et al.* (2013) noted that even though there was no gender difference in the adherence to anti-hypertension drugs, the reasons behind why *did* differ. For men, those who were concerned about their Body Mass Index and sexual functioning were less likely to adhere to treatment. For women it was those who were dissatisfied with their health and social care provider and those showing depressive symptoms that did not adhere to treatment.

Social support: family and friends

Individuals living with a spouse or relative (Lorenc and Branthwaite, 1993) or with close social relationships (Doherty *et al.*, 1983) are, in general, more likely to adhere to medical advice than isolated people. For example, Bovbjerg *et al.* (1995) found that men whose wives were supportive were more likely to stick to a prescribed change in diet than those whose families were unsupportive. Similarly, Sherbourne *et al.* (1992) reported that adherence to advice about managing diabetes was better in individuals who had more social support. In a study that manipulated levels of support, Tanner and Feldman (1997) found that individuals whose significant other (e.g. partner) received supportive counselling were more likely to attend subsequent appointments.

However, Sherwood (1983) found that haemodialysis patients were most likely to comply if their families were neither too over- nor under-involved emotionally. This suggests that social support is vital but that a measure of independence may also be important.

Personality and beliefs

As with findings about age and adherence, there is little evidence for links between adherence and personality in the general population. In fact, some studies have clearly demonstrated that the same individual will show different levels of compliance in differing situations (Lutz *et al.*, 1983; Orme and Binik, 1989). However, some specific groups do demonstrate differences. Individuals with obsessive-compulsive disorder (OCD) are, perhaps unsurprisingly, more compliant. Kabat-Zin and Chapman-Waldrop (1988) found that people with high scores on an OCD scale were more likely to stick to an 8-week stress-reduction programme than those with low scores.

Christensen *et al.* (1997) used a scale of cynical hostility (which measures personality characteristics such as suspiciousness, anger and resentfulness) to assess haemodialysis patients. Those with high scores were less likely to adhere to advice on diet and medication. Lack of adherence is also characteristic of individuals with avoidance-based coping mechanisms (Sherbourne *et al.*, 1992). Avoidant individuals employ strategies such as 'something will turn up' and 'it might simply disappear' (see also external locus of control, Chapter 3).

Unlike stable personality traits, some temporary changes in an individual's emotional state do appear to be linked to increased or reduced compliance. Optimistic patients are more likely to follow treatment advice (Leedham *et al.*,

1995) whereas depressed patients are less likely to (Carney *et al.*, 1995). Similarly, Cipher *et al.* (2002) investigated compliance in patients suffering chronic pain. They found that those who suppressed negative emotions (such as anger) showed greater adherence to treatment whereas those with amplified negative emotions were less compliant.

However, more recent research is beginning to find some patterns. Axelsson *et al.* (2011) examined how differing personality types might affect adherence in a Swedish sample. A total of 749 patients, all with chronic disease completed questionnaires that measured their personality on aspects like extraversion and neuroticism alongside their adherence to treatment. Those who scored high on the neuroticism scale were much *less* likely to adhere whilst those who scored high on agreeableness and conscientiousness were *more* likely to adhere. The effect of neuroticism was also a predictor for non-adherence to a trial of *Gingko biloba* for memory loss and dementia in a cohort of older adults in California (Jerant *et al.*, 2011).

Elements of personality can also affect adolescents' adherence to diabetic treatment.

RESEARCH IN BRIEF

Wheeler *et al.* (2012) Personality traits as predictors of adherence in adolescents with type I diabetes.

Aim: To investigate the role of personality factors in adolescents adhering to good practice linked to having type I diabetes

Method: They examined 28 adolescents with type I diabetes in terms of personality type and adherence to things like blood glucose monitoring, insulin administration and diet.

Results: Similar to the findings above, Neuroticism and Conscientiousness had the biggest effect on adherence. The table below shows some of the aspects of personality that were linked to adherence.

Adherence to...	Elements of personality that predicted adherence
Insulin administration	Low levels of anger and depression plus higher levels of self-discipline
Diet	Low levels of impulsiveness and high levels of self-discipline
Exercise	High levels of assertiveness

In more general terms those with low levels of Neuroticism were *more likely* to adhere to insulin administration. Those with higher levels of Extraversion tended to adhere to exercise regimes more often. Those with high levels of Conscientiousness were more likely to adhere to insulin administration and diet.

Conclusion: Therefore, it would seem that when an illness has a range of behaviours that need adhering to, not one single type of personality can predict adherence but different elements *within* a personality might add together to explain it.

Personal beliefs do seem to be important when it comes to adherence. According to the health belief model, patients are more likely to adhere to advice when they:

- **Perceive themselves to be vulnerable**: e.g. a woman recognizing that breast cancer could run in her own family so she should follow advice to attend screening.
- **Perceive their condition to be serious**: e.g. having known several women who have died of cervical cancer encouraging a woman to respond to an invitation to have a smear test.
- **Believe that their health will benefit from adherence**: e.g. an asthmatic who knows that using their preventer will improve their breathing is more likely to follow guidance to do so.
- **Perceive few barriers to adherence**: e.g. a patient who believes that a dietary programme can be maintained so is more likely to stick to it.
- **Have their behaviour prompted by a cue to action**: e.g. receiving a reminder to attend an appointment may encourage an individual to go for a dental check-up.

An example of these factors in action comes from Meichenbaum and Turk (1987) who observed that people are less likely to follow advice when they judge that barriers (such as side-effects) exceed possible benefits (such as long-term health). This perception may be enhanced by an awareness of the reality that conscientious adherence can lead to more side-effects (Kaplan and Simon, 1990).

The theory of planned behaviour suggests that patients are more likely to adhere to advice when:

- they have a positive attitude towards the behaviour required by compliance
- the subjective norms support compliance
- they therefore perceive themselves to be in control of their behaviour
- they intend to comply with the advice.

Again, evidence supports this idea. For example, Horne and Weinman (2002) investigated adherence to preventer medication by asthmatics. They found that individuals who had doubts about the necessity of the medication and concerns about its side-effects (indicating a negative attitude towards compliance) were less likely to adhere.

Finally, we explore the ideas of self-efficacy and locus of control. Self-efficacy is an individual's confidence in his or her own ability to perform a behaviour. When a patient is confident that they can comply with advice, they are more likely to do so. For example, an asthmatic patient who believes they are able to use their inhaler competently is more likely to adhere to advice about usage than an individual who does not feel they can use it successfully. Research supports this prediction. McAuley (1993) reported that individuals with high self-efficacy were more likely to have stuck to an aerobic exercise programme for 4 months.

Locus of control refers to whether the individual believes that they are responsible for their own health outcomes (internal locus of control) or that their health is governed by factors beyond their control (external locus of control). Individuals with a high internal locus of control feel that they have personal choice so are more likely to follow advice because this enables them to exert their control over the situation. For example, Koski-Jannes (1994) found that those participants on an abstinence programme for alcoholics who had a strong internal locus of control were more likely to maintain their abstinence.

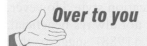

Over to you

You have been asked to write a brief report about why individuals might not adhere to treatment by your manager. They want to know **two** factors that can affect adherence. Write them a brief report using evidence to back up your claims.

KEY POINTS

1　There are many explanations as to why patients do not adhere to treatment including a Cognitive Model a Behavioural Model.

2　Theories of memory like the multistore model and levels of processing can also explain why people remember or forget details about the treatments they are currently undertaking.

3　There are individual factors that can affect adherence to treatment like gender, social support, personality and locus of control.

HEALTH PRACTITIONER BEHAVIOUR AND ADHERENCE

Just as differences between patients affect adherence, so do the characteristics of different health and social care practitioners. Factors such as their communication skills, communication style, competence and gender can each affect adherence by the patient.

Communication skills

As we discussed in Chapter 2, effective communication plays a key role in good health and social care and is therefore important to adherence. DiMatteo *et al.* (1986) found that those doctors who were most attuned to the nonverbal cues of others had more reliable patients.

In speaking to patients, doctors focus on the task of diagnosis; asking questions and obtaining sufficient information to come to a conclusion about their diagnosis or proposed treatment. Doctors may therefore be selective in the aspects of a patient's answers to which they respond. A patient, however, may be concerned about one particular symptom that has little bearing on the diagnosis, so is ignored. As a consequence, the patient may conclude that the doctor is not listening to them or is not concerned, and therefore may feel unsatisfied with their treatment. This dissatisfaction can lead to reduced compliance. Furthermore, patients may cease to attend to the doctor's instructions, further reducing the possibility of compliance.

Elsewhere we have discussed various roles for emotion – its impact on patients' memory and on communication. For example, we have discussed the benefits of a more emotionally focused communication style. However, emotionality in the health and social care context is not always beneficial. Evidence from a study conducted by Rorer *et al.* (1988) suggests that emotionally toned information, whether it is positive or negative, is less likely to result in compliance. Patients on haemodialysis were most likely to adhere to instructions when the health and social care professional–patient relationship was maintained with emotionally neutral responses.

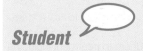

Student

Student nurse in an orthopaedic ward

Understanding the background

'I had a 70 year-old female patient on my ward that became so stressed and angry when she was told by her doctor that she would have to remain in hospital for several days following a hip replacement operation that she refused food and medication. When I approached her about this I learned that she hadn't understood why she was to stay in hospital for so long, and that she was worried who would care for her elderly husband at home. Following an explanation from me about her expected recovery period, and a visit from her family reassuring her that her husband would be cared for, she settled on the ward.'

Improving patient attention to and understanding of medical information

Improving attention

In order for patients to comply, they must be aware of and be able to hear, or see and read, the message intended for them. Some ways to ensure that this is achieved are suggested as follows:

- Get the message noticed.
- Use verbal warnings, e.g. 'Danger' Hazard' or 'Caution'.
- Use colour, bold, size, fonts, borders, prominent position.
- Use graphic symbols.
- Use attention-raising gimmicks, e.g. flip books for putting on condoms.
- Make the message legible or audible. In print, use good contrast, size and spacing to ensure readability and avoid writing text in capitals.

Improving understanding

Ley and Llewelyn (1995) have identified two aspects of spoken communication that help to improve patient understanding, so are implicated in adherence:

- Important points should be stressed – according to Ley (1972) this increases recall by 15 per cent.
- Information should be simplified, using shorter words and sentences – Bradshaw *et al.* (1975) report that this increased recall by 13 per cent.

In addition to suggesting ways to increase adherence by improving spoken communication, Ley and Llewelyn (1995) also recommended the use of written communication. There are several reasons for this:

- Even when good practice in spoken communication is evident, non-compliance may still be a problem (Ley, 1988).
- The content of written material can be designed to maximize understandability and memorability.
- Written material can be used as a source of reference for patients.
- Patients want printed information – e.g. Gibbs *et al.* (1990) found that 97 per cent of a sample of British patients would like to receive written information about their medication.

Of course, just because patients demonstrate a desire for written material does not mean that supplying it will necessarily lead to improved adherence. The information must still be read, understood and followed. From a series of studies conducted in Britain, Gibbs *et al.* (1987) have reported that 88 per cent of 117 patients taking penicillin or non-steroidal anti-inflammatory drugs (NSAIDs) read leaflets about their drugs and 97 per cent of a sample of 349 patients taking NSAIDs, beta-adrenoceptor antagonists or inhaled bronchodilators claimed to have read their leaflets (Gibbs *et al.*, 1989). These figures are encouragingly high. Estimates from Ley (1988) for US samples have found variable percentages of patients claiming to have read leaflets about their medication (49–97 per cent) but fewer (22–57 per cent) kept the leaflets and referred to them.

Finally, understanding may relate not only to understanding 'what' is required but also understanding 'how'. Skills training is designed to help patients to make appropriate judgements and perform required behaviours. McCulluch *et al.* (1983) used skills training to help patients with insulin-dependent diabetes to manage their diet correctly. The patients were offered menus from which they had to select appropriate foods and quantities, and received immediate feedback from a dietician about their choices. Within 7 days a greater improvement was apparent in the dietary management of patients in the skills training group than in those receiving information or education only.

The effect of familiarity and cues to behaviour change

Even if patients have read warnings and understood them, they may still ignore them, especially if the message is very familiar. For example, research conducted at the Centre for Behavioural Research in Cancer (1992) found that individuals who had been smoking for longer were less likely to be able to recall warning messages on cigarette packets than were smokers who had acquired the habit more recently (although contrast this finding with that of MacKinnon and Fenaughty (1993). One explanation for the apparent habituation to warning messages is offered by Breznitz (1984). According to Breznitz, the credibility of the message is reduced because the smoker has evidence that it is a 'false alarm' since they are able to smoke one, then progressively many cigarettes without any clear signal that the behaviour is damaging. Research conducted by Borland and Naccarella (1991) supports this view, as older smokers are less likely to attribute the cause of smoking-related illnesses to their habit.

Somewhat surprisingly, not even actual alarms such as accidents or injuries seem to act as effective cues to change behaviour. For example, Bragg (1973) found that seat belt use was not affected by the occurrence of injuries in car accidents (contrast this finding with the evidence for the importance of cues to action according to the health belief model).

Improving patients' memory for medical information

In order to recall information, it must be attended to and, preferably understood, so attempts to make material more obvious or comprehensible will also improve memory for that information. In addition, based on the research discussed previously, the following recommendations can be made that would specifically improve the likelihood of patients remembering information presented to them about health matters.

- Present information in small amounts (to enable chunking in STM).
- Ensure information can be understood (to allow deep processing to occur).

- Present key information first (so that the primacy effect ensures that it is transferred to LTM) – Ley (1972) showed that this improved recall by 36 per cent.
- Repeat key information (to improve rehearsal and transfer to LTM) – Ley (1979) and Bertakis (1977) showed that repetition increased recall and satisfaction.
- Present information sufficiently slowly, or with gaps, to avoid displacement and do not ask questions immediately after providing information.

Houts *et al.* (1998) found that the provision of cues in the form of pictographs helped to improve recall for spoken medical instructions. The participants, students from a remedial reading class, were tested on their ability to remember a list of 38 instructions for managing fever and 50 for managing a sore mouth. They recalled only 14 per cent of the verbal instructions without any cues but 85 per cent when assisted by the visual memory cues.

Encouraging patients to follow advice that they understand and remember

Even if we are able to provide information that patients can understand and recall, this will not automatically lead to adherence – they must take steps to actually follow that advice. For example, in patients with diabetes, improving understanding through education does not guarantee better control of blood glucose or reduce hospitalization (Goodall and Halford, 1991; Shillitoe, 1988). The following sections consider ways to make acting on advice more likely.

Applying the behavioural model: reinforcing adherence

The processes of operant conditioning can be used to increase adherence. Patients can be provided with cues to trigger appropriate behaviours and such responses can be rewarded with positive reinforcement. Some reinforcers may be intrinsic, i.e. internal to the individual – such as feeling good about losing weight – whilst others are extrinsic, i.e. from an external source – such as praise from the health and social care professional. Hegel *et al.* (1992) successfully used positive reinforcers, shaping and self-management with haemodialysis patients to improve their adherence to dietary advice with requirements. They suggested that such strategies may be at least as effective at gaining adherence as cognitive approaches – and easier to implement.

Examples of cues for adherence:

- postal, telephone or email reminders for appointments
- pill calendars or packets marked with days of the week
- visual reminders such as hand written notes

Examples of positive reinforcers:

- feeling fitter
- money
- stickers for children attending dental appointments.

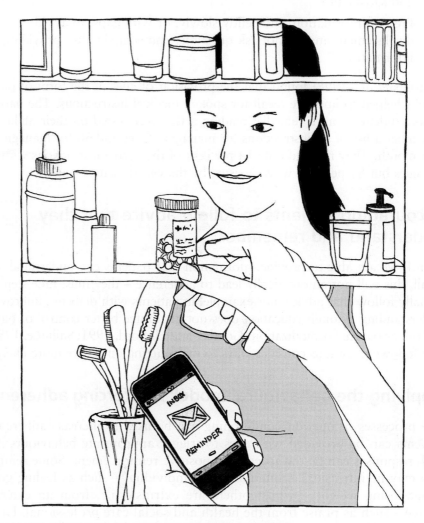

How can your patients remind themselves to take their medication?

The employment of a token economy is a way to ensure that positive reinforcers are contingent, and therefore effective. Patients are rewarded for adherence with tokens that can be exchanged later for desirable items or opportunities (such as watching television).

The effectiveness of incentives can also be interpreted using the behavioural model. An incentive acts to 'suggest' the possibility of a reward, making the benefits of reinforcement desirable. Incentives can therefore act both as cues to trigger behaviour and as immediate (i.e. contingent) intrinsic reinforcers. An example of incentives in action would be the use of contracts between patients and health and social care professionals, for instance in gaining compliance from adolescents with insulin-dependent diabetes. The contract both provides a cue – a reminder of the action to be performed – and acts to generate a positive reinforcer – the satisfaction of knowing that you have fulfilled the contract.

Self-monitoring can also act as an incentive strategy, providing cues and intrinsic rewards. This has been used successfully by Wing *et al.* (1986) to assist patients with diabetes. The patients are equipped with the skills to monitor blood glucose levels accurately and use this information to regulate carefully with injections. They then reinforce themselves for improved blood glucose control and for adherence such as eating a good diet and taking exercise.

Enhancing personal relevance

One disadvantage of supplying patients with pre-printed material is that it must be general. This is problematic because patients are more likely to comply if the advice they are given is personally tailored so that they can see how it is relevant to them. This requires health and social care professionals to individualize instructions and to try to fit programmes (such as diet, exercise or taking of medication) into the individual's daily routine.

Removing barriers to adherence

If the treatment programme can be kept short and simple, patients are more likely to adhere to it. For example, Haynes *et al.* (1987) found that patients were more likely to stick to a medication regimen if the doses were less frequent. The difficulty of organizing or remembering is reduced, removing a barrier and increasing adherence.

Enhancing social support

Adherence can be improved by encouraging the patient's family or friends to become involved in understanding the treatment. Morisky (1983) found that hypertensive patients benefited from enhanced social support. Patients allocated to interventions involving home visits that aimed to increase social support were more likely to have survived 5 years later.

Encouraging self-efficacy

Individuals who believe that they can adhere are more likely to do so, so setting patients achievable goals should improve adherence. Kalichman *et al.* (2002) found that self-efficacy with regards to 'condom skills' predicted the use of condoms by male and female adolescents on a substance abuse treatment programme. However, Norman *et al.* (2003) found that, although parents of children with amblyopia (squint) who had higher self-efficacy were more motivated to comply with eye-patching, in fact, only perceived vulnerability and response costs (barriers) were significant predictors of adherence.

IMPROVING ADHERENCE – WHAT IS CURRENTLY BEING USED IN HEALTH AND SOCIAL CARE SETTINGS?

There have been many attempts at improving adherence in patients with many having a focus on the patient doing all of the work. Both traditional and more information technology based methods are used with an emphasis on now 'reminding' the patient of their duties rather than expecting them to remember everything about their own treatment regime without 'prompts'. This next section looks at a variety of techniques that have been used.

One way to improve adherence could be to call people to remind them of their treatment regime and give further advice if necessary. Castle, Cunningham and Marsh (2012) examined an Interactive Voice Response Telephone Call (IVR) and its effects on antidepressive drug adherence. One month after being prescribed with an antidepressive, 39 020 people received an IVR. The IVR was a pre-recorded series of scripts that would give information about things like side-effects, adherence with an opportunity for the person to be transferred to a 'real life' consultant. The person receiving the call did not know to expect one and they could answer any questions either by speaking or typing in answers via their telephone keypad. A total of over 11 000 patients did pick up the call of which just fewer than 300 then chose the option to chat with the 'real life' consultant. Adherence rates were analyzed for the not reached group, the reached group who did not request the 'real life' consultant and those who did. Initially, the data look promising as adherence rates were highest in those who did seek a 'real life' consultation followed by those who picked up the call with the not reached group being last. However, on closer analysis, Castle and the team noted that age was a confounding variable. In all three groups, adherence increased with age, so older patients were more likely to adhere *irrespective* of which group they were in. Therefore, IVR may be useful for some older patients but those who are younger may need a different approach to improving adherence.

Use of text messaging

As the number of mobile phones increasingly grows, health and social care providers may be able to use these to improve adherence to treatment via simple text reminders. Lewis *et al.* (2013) reported on a scheme that sent tailored text messages to people currently undergoing HIV treatment. After being assessed prior to receiving text messages, the patients received reminder texts, answered weekly adherence texts and for those who adhered to treatment they received tailored messages like 'He shoots! He scores! Perfect med adherence. Great job!' (p. 250). For those found to be non-adherent they were sent reminder texts like 'Stop, drop and pop. Take your meds now!' (p. 250). The patients reported being very receptive to the text messaging system and appreciated the messages. The adherence to medication (self-reported) improved significantly during the 3 months receiving the texts (especially those who had begun the study not adhering to treatment). Objective measures of adherence like viral load confirmed that these patients had been adhering to treatment.

Letters

Even with information technology dominating people's lives, Zhang and Fish (2012) examined whether a simple letter through the post may improve adherence to a variety of treatments in a health and social care setting. They also wanted to investigate whether different types of treatment were affected in the same way via a reminder letter. Adult patients were followed to check for adherence rates to a variety of health issues like colonoscopies, general X-rays, vaccines and general eye tests for diabetics. A first reminder letter was sent out 1 month after the appropriate time frame for treatment for urgent cases (2 months for non-urgent). If these were not responded to then the second letter was sent out 1 month after the first. Table 6.1 shows the adherence rates for a variety of treatments followed in the study:

Table 6.1 The adherence rates for a variety of treatments followed in the study				
Treatment	**No reminder**	**One letter reminder**	**Two letter reminder**	**Non-adherence**
Colonoscopy	35	11	14	45
Mammogram	57	16	5	34
Cardiac testing	11	5	0	4
Ultrasound	55	7	1	5

Note: Numbers refer to number of patients.

As can be seen, for some of the treatments above, no reminder was necessary. However, for all of the treatments listed above, people did respond to a letter reminding them of the importance of the treatment which led to them attending the relevant health clinic. From the data above, those sent a second letter that required a colonoscopy, responded well with another 14 people coming forward. The high levels of non-adherence to both the colonoscopy and mammogram highlight that some people simply do *not* respond to reminders. Research into why these people do not respond needs to be conducted.

Memory Intervention

A recent development has been created by Insel *et al.* (2013) to aid adherence to antihypertensive drugs. Previous studies had been noted by this research team to just focus on one aspect of adherence (e.g. just understanding how many pills to take). Insel *et al.* have proposed a multifaceted approach to improving adherence through *cognitive* tasks (note the plural). The following is part of the model that they believe will improve adherence:

- Emphasize routine – have medication in same place and same time each day or each time it has to be taken.
- Develop cues – for example, have a pill pot on the breakfast table in full view rather than in a box in a drawer.
- Elaborate the action – for example, get the patient to shake the bottle before taking the pills to make it more memorable so they don't take a repeat dose immediately.
- Do it now – as soon as a cue is present take the pills there and then – a 5 second delay can cause forgetting and non-adherence.
- Implementation intentions – make it all specific, so rather than thinking 'around breakfast time I will take my pills' get them to think 'with my first cup of tea of the day I will take my pills'.
- Teach – ask – wait – ask again – wait – ask again: this allows them to rehearse intentions and leaving a sufficient gap at the second 'wait' (as long as 15 minutes) can help improve memory for intention according to Insel *et al*.

It will be intriguing to see if the system does improve adherence rates to antihypertensive drugs.

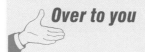

Over to you

The NHS have asked you for your help – over £150 million worth of drugs are returned to pharmacies each year (many through non-adherence). They want to reduce this figure. Produce a report highlighting *at least two ways* in which adherence could be improved in patients. Use evidence to strengthen the arguments in your report.

KEY POINTS:

1 There are a number of ways in which adherence to treatment may be improved including communication skills, improving attention and improving memory.

2 Contemporary techniques to help improve adherence to treatments include text messaging, telephone calls and memory interventions.

CONCLUSIONS

Patients receiving medical treatment do not necessarily follow the advice they have been given. This may be the case even when they are told that they are seriously ill. Being afraid, having a complex medication regimen, suffering side-effects or having to find time to make a change in lifestyle all tend to reduce adherence to medical advice. Patients who are in pain or who believe themselves to be very ill are more likely to adhere as are those who have good social support. Some factors, such as age, gender and personality, have few consistent effects on adherence. Health and social care practitioners themselves can also affect patients' adherence through their communication skills, communication style, competence and gender.

Non-adherence may be explained in a number of different ways: through the effects of factors that act as rewards (such as recovery) or punishment (such as side-effects), or by a lack of understanding or recall by patients. Dissatisfied patients are also less likely to adhere to instructions. Health behaviour models additionally suggest that individuals who perceive few barriers to adherence, think that they will benefit, have cues to trigger the following of advice, have a positive attitude to treatment, believe that they are in control of their own behaviour and intend to comply with advice are more likely to do so.

The findings of research in this area provide a range of suggestions for ways to improve adherence to medical advice. Techniques aim to increase attention to, and memory and understanding of the advice given, enhance personal relevance of information, remove barriers to following the advice, increase social support and raise the patient's belief that they are able to adhere.

RAPID RECAP

1 What are the differences between the Behavioural and Cognitive models of compliance?

2 Explain how personality might affect adherence to treatment.

3 Outline two ways in which we could improve adherence to treatment.

If you have difficulty with any of the questions, read through the section again to refresh your understanding before moving on.

KEY REFERENCE

Other references are listed on the supporting website.

Wheeler, K., Wagaman, A. and McCord, D. (2012) Personality traits as predictors of adherence in adolescents with type I diabetes. *Journal Child Adolescnt Psychiatric Nursing* 25 (2): 66–74

CHAPTER 7

STRESS

LEARNING OBJECTIVES

By the end of this chapter you should be able to:

- discuss biological and psychological explanations of stress

- describe research into the links between stress and health

- describe sources of stressors for patients and health and social care professionals

- identify biological, social and psychological factors that can increase an individual's experience of stress

- identify ways in which stress can affect social behaviour and performance

- describe and evaluate stress management strategies that could be used by patients and health and social care professionals.

THE CONCEPT OF STRESS

Stress is a reaction, both physical and psychological, to circumstances that are perceived to be negative and threatening to the individual. The elements of the situation that provoke such a response are called stressors. Some kinds of stimuli, under particular circumstances, may become stressful. Stressors could affect us in one of two ways:

- Physiologically by affecting body functioning such as altering pulse rate, blood pressure and the immune system or by changing hormone levels.

- Psychologically through sensitivity changes in cognitive functioning and emotions such as fear or anger.

Some of these responses are adaptive; they help us to respond to potential dangers. However, they evolved to protect us when our environment was different from that in which we now live. The stress responses that helped primitive humans avoid being eaten by fast-moving predators are of little help to a stressed patient awaiting surgery or an overworked physiotherapist faced with a patient list so long as to be beyond capacity. Neither would have much to gain by being able to run fast!

FACTORS INVOLVED IN THE EXPLANATION OF STRESS

Stressors can be categorized as either internal (individual) or external (environmental). These two classes of stressor can also operate in combination.

Internal factors and stress

Some stressors are internal, that is they originate within us. The sensation of anxiety can arise without any obvious stimulus from the outside yet it can make us stressed. Such feelings may be irrational and without an apparent cause, but they can be very stressful. A range of thoughts and feelings may be stressful. Worrying about things that may never happen, such as fretting about not waking up from an anaesthetic or finding a malignant lump. Pain is also an internal source of stress; a nagging headache or chronic back pain could act as a stressor. Similarly, being ill or unable to sleep are internal experiences that can induce stress. An individual who lies in bed fretting about being tired the next morning because they cannot fall asleep is experiencing stress even though there may be no external trigger for their sleeplessness.

External factors and stress

In approaches that focus on external factors, stress is seen as something that happens to an individual rather than within them. Stress arises when levels of stressors, such as the pressures of work become too high. Thus physical situations such as crowding or noise, and social situations such as missing a loved one, or being forced to engage with unpleasant or frightening people, is stressful. Being a new patient on a ward could therefore present external stressors. Life events theory identifies key occurrences, such as changing jobs that are stressful.

The incidence of stress among health and social care professionals is known to be high (e.g. Borrill *et al.*, 1998). Some reasons for this include lack of clarity about roles, conflict, excess work demands and lack of control over work. Such factors are external to the individual.

Interactional factors and stress

This approach suggests that stress arises from an interaction between the environment and the individual's response to it. Importantly, it emphasizes the psychological factors that allow some people to cope with more stressful environments than others.

Antagonistic
Paired systems that
work in opposition,
such as parts of the
nervous system that
increase or decrease
arousal

Endocrine system
Bodily communication
route composed of
glands releasing
hormones that travel
via the blood to target
organs

Hormones
Chemicals released by
endocrine glands into
the bloodstream that
acts as a
communication
system in the body

Adrenal medulla
The inner part of the
adrenal glands, which
releases the hormone
adrenaline
(epinephrine)

Catecholamines
A group of
neurotransmitters
with a similar
chemical structure to
adrenaline that
includes dopamine
and noradrenaline
(norepinephrine)

Lazarus's appraisal model incorporates such an interaction. It suggests that the way an individual perceives and responds to a stimulus (i.e. copes) determines their experience of stress. When the individual judges their resources to be inadequate in comparison to their perception of the challenge, there are emotional and physiological responses and they feel stressed. This helps to explain why the relationship between a potential stressor and the stress an individual suffers is not a simple one. People may differ in the way they appraise, and therefore tackle, the demands of a situation as well as in their personal resources.

For example, one patient may experience a forthcoming procedure as something that will be unpleasant but that they can endure whereas another may anticipate that the consequences will be intolerable. Thus the second individual, will experience stress as they appraise the situation to be difficult (or impossible) to cope with.

THEORIES OF STRESS

Physiological explanations of stress

The physiological response to stress is mediated by two bodily systems. One, the autonomic nervous system, is composed of two approximately antagonistic sub-systems, the sympathetic and parasympathetic branches. The autonomic nervous system acts rapidly to stimulate physiological changes, such as breathing and heart rate, as well as affecting the second element, the endocrine system. The endocrine system provides a slower communication route through the body, using hormones released in response to signals from nerves or from other glands.

Autonomic nervous system

In an emergency, the sympathetic branch of the autonomic nervous system responds quickly, preparing for 'fight or flight'. The sympathetic nervous system also sends impulses to the endocrine system, which responds by releasing hormones that enhance the preparation for action. This mechanism, which links the sympathetic nervous system to the adrenal medulla, is called the sympathetic adrenal medullary system. Although the sympathetic response is very fast, allowing us to respond quickly to an emergency, its effects are short-lived.

Endocrine system

The effects of the endocrine system are slower but longer lasting. Adrenaline (epinephrine) is released from the adrenal medulla in response to stressors, as are related neurotransmitters (catecholamines) including noradrenaline (norepinephrine). This elevated level of catecholamines during stress may be responsible for some of the effects of stress on health, such as hardening of the arteries. In addition, the adrenal cortex releases corticosteroid hormones.

The general adaptation syndrome

Selye (1947) described the body's response to stress and began to explore the links between the nervous system, the endocrine system and illness. He induced stress in rats using stressors including heat and fatigue. The rats showed the same physiological responses regardless of the nature of the stressor; they had enlarged adrenal glands, shrunken lymph glands and stomach ulcers. Selye proposed that the body responded to any stressor by mobilizing itself for action, a response he called the general adaptation syndrome. This response has evolved to help the individual to deal with emergency situations such as fleeing physical danger. Selye identified three phases to the body's response to stress through which an individual passes if a stressor persists over time:

- **Alarm reaction**: the body's mechanisms for dealing with danger are activated.
- **Resistance stage**: the person struggles to cope with the stress and the body attempts to return to its previous physiological state.
- **Exhaustion stage**: if the stressor persists and the body cannot return to its previous state, physical resources become depleted, eventually leading to collapse.

A great deal more is now known about the precise mechanisms controlling the response to stress than Selye first observed as described below.

The sympathetic adrenal medullary system

In the initial response to a potentially threatening stimulus the sympathetic branch of the autonomic nervous system prepares the body quickly for action. The sympathetic response also causes the release of hormones, adrenaline and noradrenaline, from the adrenal medulla. The combined effect of the sympathetic adrenal medullary system ensures that the body is physically prepared to counter the environmental threat, for instance by fighting or fleeing. The sympathetic adrenal medullary system therefore controls responses to acute (short-term) stressors. The effects of the sympathetic response, which resembles the action of adrenaline, is illustrated in the flow chart (Figure 7.1).

The hypothalamic–pituitary–adrenocortical axis

If the stressor is not removed the body responds differently, reducing levels of adrenaline and noradrenaline and increasing levels of three other hormones:

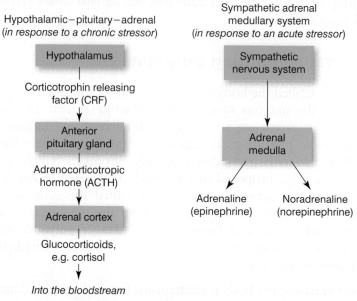

Figure 7.1   The effects of stressors

- Cortisol breaks down fatty tissue, releasing soluble fats and stimulating the release of glucose from the liver so that the muscles can obtain more energy from the blood.
- Aldosterone increases blood pressure, maintaining the body ready for action.
- Thyroxine increases the body's metabolic rate. This means that the stressed person can extract energy from food more quickly. Thyroxine also increases the rate at which food travels through the gut, allowing energy to be quickly obtained from the food currently in the gut.

The release of corticosteroids such as cortisol from the adrenal cortex is controlled by another hormone, adrenocorticotrophic hormone (ACTH) from the pituitary gland. ACTH is in turn secreted in response to the release of corticotrophin-releasing factor (CRF). CRF is a **peptide** released by the paraventricular nucleus, a region of the hypothalamus. Soendergaard and Theorell (2003) reported raised cortisol levels in refugees, particularly when they were experiencing distress in significant others (such as close friends or relatives) and excessive demands on everyday life.

Injection of CRF into the brain produces responses similar to those associated with **aversive** situations, supporting the belief that some aspects of the stress response are caused by CRF. For example, Swerdlow *et al.* (1986) found that CRF increased the startle response shown by rats to a loud noise. This link between the hypothalamus, the pituitary gland and the adrenal cortex is referred to as the hypothalamic-pituitary-adrenocortical axis and can trigger the release of corticosteroids to minor but unpredictable changes. If these are not threatening, the response diminishes as cortisol feeds back to

Peptide
A small protein

Aversive
Something that is perceived to be unpleasant

the hypothalamus and pituitary gland to limit further releases of CRF and ACTH. If, however, the situation is sustained (in the case of a chronic stressor) the action of the hypothalamic-pituitary-adrenocortical axis is maintained by the forebrain (see Figure 7.1).

If the stressor is severe and prolonged, exhaustion may result. Examples of such stressors include being hunted, tortured or working in a high-demand profession, such as the health and social care professions. Exhaustion occurs when the body's supplies of energy are used up. This may ultimately result in collapse and sometimes death. Furthermore, these systems are adapted to protect us from environmental stressors present in our evolutionary history, such as being chased by a sabre-toothed tiger, but we are now exposed to rather different problems, such as working shifts or talking to bereaved relatives.

One consequence of this biological endowment is that our coping strategies fail to deal effectively with the demands of modern living, causing chronic sympathetic adrenal medullary activation rather than leading to hypothalamic–pituitary–adrenocortical activity. The effects, such as prolonged elevation of pulse rate and blood pressure, put strain on the cardiovascular system with, perhaps, the consequence of increased levels of cardiovascular disorders. Where coping is less effective, for example because control is limited, another characteristic of modern living, hypothalamic–pituitary–adrenocortical activity will be triggered. Where such stressors are chronic, immunosuppression may result as corticosteroids such as cortisol affect immune functioning.

The two systems, the sympathetic adrenal medullary system and the hypothalamic–pituitary–adrenocortical axis have been represented here as independent although, in reality, they are not. The neurotransmitters noradrenaline and serotonin, natural endorphins and the hormone cortisol all act as intermediaries between the two systems.

> **Immuno-suppression**
> Reduced capacity of the body to fight disease due to deactivation of the immune response

Stress and the immune system

The immune system is a collection of structures and mechanisms that our bodies use to fight off disease. The lymphatic system consists of branching vessels that drain tissue fluid containing micro organisms away from the cells of the body back into the blood. Various kinds of white blood cells called lymphocytes are responsible for different aspects of the immune response (Table 7.1). Changes in levels of these cells and their products (immunoglobulins) can be measured and related to levels of stress (Pitts and Phillips, 1998).

According to Cooper *et al.* (1988), stress causes or exacerbates all of Britain's top 20 fatal illnesses. High cortisol levels resulting from prolonged stress are associated with allergic responses; so allergic conditions such as eczema and asthma can be aggravated by prolonged stress. Rheumatoid arthritis, an autoimmune disorder causing painful inflammation of the joints, is also worsened by stress (Zautra, 1998). Here, the effects of stress are

Table 7.1 Roles of different types of lymphocyte	
Cell type	**Immunological role**
B lymphocyte	Multiply in response to specific infections and produce antibodies (proteins called immunoglobulins) that bind to antigens on the cell surface of invading micro-organisms, thereby labelling them for destruction
T lymphocyte	Recognize, engulf and destroy body cells that have been infected, for example, by a virus; therefore tend to multiply during illness
Natural killer (NK) cell	Selectively target and destroy suspect cells, including cancerous cells

indirect, resulting from physiological changes that occur in response to stress. In other situations, stress directly affects health, impairing our ability to fight disease. For example, bereavement (Schleifer *et al.*, 1983), marital disruption (Kiecolt-Glaser and Glaser, 1986) and students' examinations (Kiecolt-Glaser *et al.*, 1994) all cause reduced immune functioning.

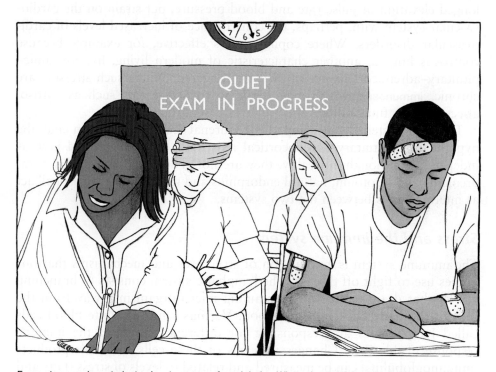

Exam stress makes students slow to recover from injuries. What other stressors do students have?

Saline solution
Salt water used in place of an active solution in an experiment

In addition to observing the effect of natural or experimental stressors on health, researchers can also test the effects of stress upon immune functioning when infection is induced. Cohen *et al.* (1993) used a nasal drip to administer either a cold virus or saline solution. The participants were then quarantined and completed measures of their stress levels. Outcome was assessed by observing both infection (multiplication of the cold virus) and clinical disease (symptoms of a cold). Participants with high stress ratings were more likely to become infected and to develop symptoms.

In a subsequent study, Cohen *et al.* (1998) found that the risk of infection increased progressively with the duration of exposure to a stressor. A parallel effect can be demonstrated for the rate of wound healing. Students are 40 per cent slower to recover from a standardized mechanical injury during exam time, when they are most stressed, than during vacations (Marucha *et al.*, 1998).

Recent research suggests that, whilst long-term stress induces immunosuppression, resulting in an increased risk of infection and disease, short-term stress may trigger an enhancement of the immune response. In psychologically challenging situations, such as public speaking or confrontational role play, increases in natural killer (NK) cells and other lymphocytes has been observed (Evans, 1998).

The explanation for these differences seems to lie in the two physiological systems controlling the stress response. The sympathetic adrenal medullary system seems to be temporarily activated in short-term acute stress, an effective evolutionary response that enables organisms to mobilize resources to fight possible infection caused by injury. Such elevated responses would, however, be damaging in themselves if prolonged. In contrast, one of the functions of the hypothalamic–pituitary–adrenocortical axis, which is activated when stressors are chronic, is to induce immunosuppression.

There is also considerable evidence for a link between stress and cancer although none indicates that stress causes cancer. Animal studies, such as that of Seligman and Visintainer (1985), have found that rates of cancer in laboratory animals increase when they are stressed. Similar results have been obtained in studies of humans. Eysenck (1988) followed up nearly 400 individuals and found that death rates from cancer were higher for those who reported greater levels of stress at the start of the study.

Normally the immune system finds and destroys cancer cells before they can establish themselves as a tumour. However, if the immune system is functioning less efficiently, then cancerous cells are less likely to be eliminated. This arises because NK cell activity is consistently impaired by stress (Herbert and Cohen, 1993). Strategies such as smoking, which some people use in an attempt to reduce stress, actually make things worse by introducing carcinogens into the body.

Carcinogens
Chemicals that can cause cancer

Psychoneuroimmunology

Psychoneuroimmunology aims to find out why an individual's attitude or state of mind affects susceptibility to, or recovery from, illness. Clearly, stress can reduce immunocompetence. In addition, the way an individual thinks can improve the immune response. For example, Pettingale *et al.* (1985) found that women with breast cancer who fought their illness survived, on average, 5 years longer post-diagnosis. However, Salmon (2000) observes that such personality factors may link to better survival for entirely different reasons – a person with 'fighting spirit' may eat more or may attract better care from staff because they are perkier.

Psychoneuro-immunology
Investigates the effect of the mind on the function of the immune system and, consequently, health

Immuno-competence
The effectiveness of immune functioning

Keller *et al.* (1994) suggested that the key aim for psychoneuroimmunological research was to understand the relationship between:

- Psychological distress
- Immune system functioning
- The development of disease.

In reality, few studies investigate all three of these variables simultaneously. Ben-Eliyahu *et al.* (1991) injected rats with tumour material, tested their immune function (NK cell level) and observed the course of the disease (the occurrence of metastases) under two experimental conditions (stress within 1 hour or 24 hours of the injection). They found that individuals receiving the stressor and injection together had more metastatic growth. Research such as that of Marucha *et al.* (1998), described earlier, has succeeded in demonstrating a similar three-way relationship in humans.

Metastases
Secondary cancerous growth caused by the spread of cancerous cells from an original tumour (the primary site) through the blood or lymph to other parts of the body

Life events theory

Whereas Selye's model emphasizes the physiological changes associated with stress, the life events model (Holmes and Rahe, 1967) attempts to link stressful events to the incidence of stress.

Holmes and Rahe initially developed a list of potentially stressful life events on which an individual could derive a score by counting the number of stressful events that had happened to them in the last year. These included minor occurrences such as 'a vacation' or 'a change in eating habits' to major traumas including 'death of a spouse' or 'personal injury or illness'. While this demonstrated links between stress and health status, it ignored differences in severity of the possible life events and was replaced by the Social Readjustment Rating Scale (SRRS) (see Table 7.2). Recent evidence suggests, however, that there is little difference in the power of the two scales to predict ill-health (Turner and Wheaton, 1995).

RESEARCH IN BRIEF

Holmes and Rahe (1967) The social readjustment rating scale

Aim: To develop a weighting system for the critical life events identified on the Scale of Recent Events.

Procedure: Records of 5000 patients were examined for life events that arose in the months preceding the onset of their illness.

Findings: Forty-three life events were found to occur often in the prescribed period. Their relative frequency was used to generate the Social Readjustment Rating Scale (SRRS). The SRRS is a list of these life events in order and weighted according to their seriousness, i.e. the relative frequency with which they were found to occur in the patients. The weightings, called life change units, can be used to calculate a score for subsequent individuals by identifying the number of significant life events that had happened to them in a specified period of time, e.g. the preceding 6 months, and adding together the value assigned to each one.

Conclusion: The SRRS can be used to predict the likelihood of a stress-related illness arising in other individuals by looking at the total of life change units. Individuals whose experiences total in excess of 300 life change units over 1 year are more likely to suffer.

Rank	Life event	Mean value	Rank	Life event	Mean value
		Table 7.2 The Social Readjustment Rating Scale			
1	Death of spouse	100	23	Son or daughter leaving home	29
2	Divorce	73	24	Trouble with in-laws	29
3	Marital separation	65	25	Outstanding personal achievement	28
4	Jail term	63	26	Wife begins or stops work	26
5	Death of close family member	63	27	Begin or end school	26
6	Personal injury or illness	53	28	Change in living conditions	25
7	Marriage	50	29	Revision of personal habits	24
8	Fired at work	47	30	Trouble with boss	23
9	Marital reconciliation	45	31	Change in work hours or conditions	20
10	Retirement	45	32	Change in residence	20
11	Change in health of family member	44	33	Change in schools	20
12	Pregnancy	40	34	Change in recreation	19
13	Sex difficulties	39	35	Change in church activities	19
14	Gain of new family member	39	36	Change in social activities	18
15	Business readjustment	39	37	Mortgage or loan less than $10 000	
16	Change in financial state	38	38	Change in sleeping habits	
17	Death of a close friend	37	39	Change in number of family get-togethers	17
18	Change to a different line of work	36	40	Change in eating habits	16
19	Change in number of arguments with spouse	35	41	Vacation	15
20	Mortgage over $10 000	31	42	Christmas	13
21	Foreclosure of mortgage or loan	30	43	Minor violations of the law	12
22	Change in responsibilities at work	29			

The SRRS includes both positive and negative events, since any deviation from the normal life pattern has the potential to be stressful. However, subsequent evidence suggested that only unpleasant events were linked to increased illness (Ross and Mirowsky, 1979).

Initial evidence supported the predictive power of the SRRS. Rahe (1968) tested 2500 servicemen prior to tours of duty. The life change units were then related to medical records at the end of the first 6 months' service. Those individuals with SRRS scores in the top 30 per cent had nearly 90 per cent more first illnesses than those individuals in the lowest 30 per cent.

Subsequent studies (e.g. Theorell *et al.*, 1975; Goldberg and Comstock, 1976), however, have not demonstrated clear relationships between stress (as indicated by the SRRS) and ill-health. This may be because ratings of life events tend to be retrospective so rely on potentially inaccurate memories. People who are ill may perceive their lives more critically, and selectively recall negative events, or may ignore them, blaming their condition on some uncontrollable factor such as genetics, thus distorting the relationship between life events and health.

Lazarus's transactional model of stress

Lazarus suggests that an individual's experience of stress is influenced by their ability to consider the effect a stressor is having upon them. Humans can evaluate events, assessing the threat, their own vulnerability and how they might cope. From this perspective, a life event is not necessarily a source of stress; the individual's evaluation of its impact is what determines stressfulness. A student who misses a deadline but has previously been up-to-date and is confident they can catch up may be less stressed by the experience than one who knows they are about to be removed from their course for persistent tardiness. It is the perception of vulnerability and lack of control that creates a stressful situation.

Lazarus and Folkman (1984) suggest that this process of determining whether a situation is threatening, challenging or harmful is one of appraisal. Our initial impression or primary appraisal of the situation generates emotions in relation to the judgement of:

- a threat, or the anticipation of harm, generates an appraisal of fear, anxiety or worry
- harm, or damage already done, generates an appraisal of disgust, disappointment, anger or sadness
- challenge, or confidence in the face of a difficult demand, generates an appraisal of anticipation or excitement.

Following the initial appraisal, a secondary appraisal is made. This is the formation of an impression about one's ability to cope with the situation. It is a consideration of the possible options, the chances of successfully employing them and whether the action will work.

In terms of a health and social care setting, Gräßel and Adabbo (2011) used the Lazarus and Folkman model to explore the potential perceived burden of individuals caring for chronically ill family members. Figure 7.2 shows the model they created based on their review.

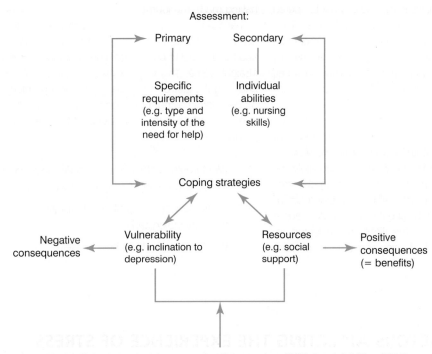

Figure 7.2   Model of the impact on homecare on the caregiver (Gräßel and Adabbo, 2011)

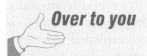

Over to you

Based on the model above, how would the following people appraise the situation: (a) a person who is a retired health and social care professional, (b) a person who has had to give up full-time work to care for their sick husband and (c) a 16 year-old who now has to look after their mum?

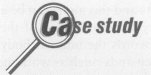

Case study

A dinosaur in a new land

Mr Jack Springwell is a 59 year-old consultant, married with three daughters. He has always worked hard and provided for his family. His wife, Eva is a teacher and since the children were teenagers has worked full time. Jack has a senior position in a small but successful engineering firm but has become irritable and moody over a period of months. His workload has increased as has the need for him to travel and be away from home. He also has to manage large numbers of emails which he finds an irritation always saying loudly that he doesn't understand why people can't just speak to each other instead of emailing. Jack is aware that new, younger members of staff have academic qualifications, such as degrees but that he has the experience. However, the strain of keeping up with new technologies and the fast pace that is now expected is taking a toll on him. He knows he is quick tempered at home and finds it almost impossible to relax. Their social circle has decreased as he is either away or often cancels arrangements made with friends at the last minute. Eva is also feeling more isolated as Jack has stopped sharing his worries with her and just constantly says he is busy at work.

This morning, Jack was waiting for an early flight to London when he suddenly started to feel light headed, short of breath and clammy. He went to the toilet and wondered how he could possibly get on the plane when he was already feeling claustrophobic. He tried to tell himself he was being ridiculous and he probably should have eaten some breakfast. He boarded the flight, which lasted 50 minutes and instead of using the time to prepare for the meeting he spent the time self-talking in his head with his eyes closed just wishing that he was on the ground. As soon as the plane landed he made his way to the door and rushed off regretting having made the journey.

Jack made it through the meeting and his presentation although it wasn't his best performance and he decided to check into a hotel instead of flying straight home. This incident had shaken him badly and was the last of a number of physical problems he had been having, but hadn't shared with colleagues or family. He therefore decided that he would go and see his GP.

1 What could Jack have done earlier to prevent the build up of conflicting responsibilities?

2 Is Jack experiencing physical problems or are they psychological?

3 What can Jack do to help himself?

Desynchronization
The separation of the circadian rhythm controlled by an internal body clock from environmental stimuli such as sunrise and sunset

Circadian rhythm
A daily cycle of activity such as sleeping and waking

Zeitgeber
A regular environmental stimulus that can set the body clock

FACTORS AFFECTING THE EXPERIENCE OF STRESS

It is possible to identify particular factors that exacerbate the stress response. Biological factors may arise as a consequence of internal stressors such as pain or external ones such as the disruption of bodily rhythms. Social factors include those situations in which the source of stress is directly related to the presence of others, for instance crowded situations or arguments. Finally, psychological factors are characteristics within us, such as our personality, that affect the way in which we respond to a potentially stressful situation.

Biological factors affecting stress

Many health and social care professionals work shifts and this alone can be a cause of stress. Changing shifts causes a temporary desynchronization of the circadian rhythm from the local zeitgebers, in other words the internal body clock is working on a different cycle from external demands (such as working hours). This disrupts many biological functions such as attention, gastrointestinal function and, most importantly, the sleep-wake cycle. Physiologically, these effects arise because the body clock continues to work on the previously established rhythm.

Cues such as daylight and other regular changes act as zeitgebers, setting the body clock to a new circadian rhythm. However, in the short term, shift workers must cope with the discrepancy between the body's needs and the immediate demands of their job. They will feel tired during the daytime but unable to fall asleep at night because their internal clock is out of tune.

Each time a shift is changed workers must readjust to a new schedule. For those on a night shift this is even more difficult, as the zeitgeber of daylight cannot help to synchronize their internal clock with the demands of their working hours. In addition to the biological disruption, other problems may arise if facilities and the family follow a daytime routine while the night-worker attempts to operate on a different pattern. Fenwick and Tausig (2000) found evidence for both family stress and health problems associated with working non-standard shifts.

Shift work is a characteristic of the health and social care profession but is detrimental to performance. Taffinder *et al.* (1998) investigated the effect of sleep deprivation on surgeons' dexterity during a simulated operation. They found that surgeons suffering overnight sleep deprivation made 20 per cent more errors, were 14 per cent slower than those who had had a full night's sleep and were more stressed.

Social factors affecting stress

Crowded places are generally experienced as stressful, being in a hospital waiting room, for example. Similarly, living in close proximity to others, in hospital accommodation or on a ward, is also stressful, especially for those who have not built up strategies for coping with high-density living. Many studies have investigated the stressful effects of crowding experimentally, on both humans and animals.

Calhoun (1962) studied the effect of restriction of space on rats. Under crowded conditions, dominant animals defended space and remained in better health than submissive ones. The latter became confined to a small area of the available space, were more aggressive and were abnormal in their reproductive behaviour and success (96 per cent of offspring died before weaning). Calhoun attributed these changes to the stress of increased social interaction. Although this study does demonstrate the negative effects of crowding on social behaviour and reproduction, it does not represent natural rat behaviour, as they would not be confined in the wild but would disperse.

Christian (1955) suggested that effects of crowding such as those described above may arise as a direct consequence of stress. Christian's social stress theory proposed that high-density existence leads to social effects that are stressful, such as competition. This would result in a stress-like response mediated by the adrenal glands (pp. 129–130). Disrupted hormone levels could then be directly responsible for the behavioural and physiological changes that have been identified.

Naturalistic observation
Systematic watching and recording of the behaviour of individuals conducting their day-to-day activities in their normal environment

To what extent are the findings from animal studies on social factors affecting stress replicated in the literature on humans? This question is difficult to answer as, although laboratory experiments into crowding are conducted, long-term investigations into the effects on humans tend to be naturalistic observations, meaning that the results are not directly comparable. The study described below investigates the payoff between frustrating and beneficial interactions with others, such as patients and staff may experience on wards or in hospital accommodation. Consider the implications of the findings for ward size.

RESEARCH IN BRIEF

Baum and Valins (1977) Architecture and social behaviour

Aim: To investigate the balance between the benefits of increased opportunities to interact as density increases and the costs of such enforced encounters.

Procedure: The perceptions and behaviour of occupants of two different types of university hall of residence were compared. The accommodation was either corridor-style or suite-style, each offering the same amount of space per individual, number of individuals per floor and the same facilities (the bathroom and lounge). They differed only in the number of other individuals sharing those facilities (either four–six in suites or 34 on corridors) and hence the number of different interpersonal encounters.

Findings: Residents in corridor-style accommodation perceived their floors to be more crowded. They were more likely to feel that they had to engage in inconvenient and unwanted social interactions and expressed a greater desire to avoid other people. Their feelings of helplessness were reflected in their social skills. They were less likely to initiate a conversation with a stranger, less able to reach a consensus after a discussion, less socially assertive and more likely to give up in a competitive game.

Conclusion: Exposure to a large number of other people, especially when the group lacks social structure, has negative consequences resulting in less sociable behaviour. The enforced, uncontrollable personal contacts experienced by the corridor residents were stressful and led to a feeling of helplessness so they tended to avoid social interactions and were less assertive in ambiguous situations because they had learned that they had little control over their social environment.

Social support
A coping strategy based on assistance from others, either direct helping or indirect encouragement. It can be received from people such as partners, family, friends and neighbours and from membership of organizations such as the church, as well as from pets

Crowding appears to reduce both liking for specific individuals and for social interaction in general. Furthermore, the effects of crowding on social interaction seem to reduce the ability to seek out others for help. Lepore *et al.* (1991) found that individuals who had high levels of social support lost this buffering effect after 8 months in crowded conditions; they no longer sought the assistance of other people as a resource in times of psychological distress. Crowding results in withdrawal; it seems to erode the social support networks that are most important in stressful situations. This finding may have implications for the rehabilitation of patients after a prolonged stay in hospital.

Evans (1979) reported that varying crowding, for instance by putting ten people in an eight-foot by 12-foot room, increased blood pressure and other physiological indicators of stress. Students living in high-density accommodation make more frequent visits to the infirmary (Baron *et al.*, 1976;

Fuller *et al.*, 1993) and report a higher level of physical illness in crowded conditions. Thus there are implications for detrimental stress-induced effects on health not only in experimental settings but in natural ones too, suggesting that health and social care environments, as potential sources of stress, can add to the burden of ill-health.

Psychological factors affecting stress

Various personality factors affect the experience of stress. For example, Firth-Cozens (1997) described the role of self-criticism in health professionals. Student doctors who displayed high self-criticism were more likely to suffer from stress and depression 10 years into their careers. Firth-Cozens observes that being able to predict which individuals are most likely to suffer from stress provides the potential for intervention and prevention. Two distinct personality types have been linked to the incidence of stress. Type A personalities are more likely to suffer from the ill-effects of stress whereas people with hardy personalities are less at risk. Locus of control is a measure of beliefs about the source of the reasons for and solutions to ill-health. Individuals with an internal locus of control may be advantaged in dealing with the effects of stress.

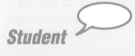

Student

Student nurse

An inexperienced eye
'I was asked to check some observations of a patient, Mr Springwell. I was asked to record his temperature, blood pressure and pulse. His pulse was irregular and his blood pressure higher than normal although his temperature was normal. It was also obvious he was easily irritated and although necessary he clearly regarded this time in the surgery as an inconvenience that was making him late for work. Without knowing much about him or his condition I remarked to the GP later that I thought if Mr Springwell didn't slow down he was going to have a heart attack or stroke and although an uninformed observation the doctor agreed with me.'

The importance of control

A person's control over a potential stressor in the environment affects the extent of the stress response it elicits. An uncontrollable noise is, for instance, more stressful than a controllable one. This relationship can be clearly demonstrated in experimental studies with animals. Seligman and Visintainer (1985) report the effects of controllable and uncontrollable shocks on the health of rats. The experimental animals were injected with live tumour cells, then exposed to electric shocks. Tumour growth was greater in the 'uncontrollable shock' condition, suggesting that stressors that cannot be controlled by the individual and are perhaps appraised as more threatening, are more detrimental to health.

Health Care Professional

General Practitioner

A flying visit

'Mr Springwell is a patient that I don't really know as he has never had occasion to visit the surgery since they moved into the area several years ago. They are an affluent, healthy family who are intelligent and well informed. He confirmed this assumption when he came to see me this morning. He told me he had recently experienced some unpleasant symptoms, which had given him reason for concern including epigastric pain and a pounding feeling in his chest. He also told me he had felt quite clammy and dizzy just prior to flying to London on a business trip.

This patient was clearly not willing to take responsibility for these symptoms, wanting a quick explanation and resolution, so he could get on with his busy life. This type of reaction is not unusual which makes it more difficult to explain that his symptoms sounded like a panic attack. To satisfy his need to rule out anything serious I decided to check his blood for a number of things including bacteria which can cause a stomach ulcer. All of his symptoms I suspected were related to work related stress as he felt there were no problems at home. In order to help someone who is feeling under stress they must be willing to admit that there may be a problem, and be willing to accept help and to help themselves. Although at the risk of alienating this patient I felt it required straight talking and I gave him my professional opinion that he was at great risk if he didn't take time out or change his lifestyle and that I was willing to help him. The first part of this was to take 2 weeks off work while we tried to get his blood pressure under control. I hoped if he agreed to this that I could meet him regularly and encourage him to talk about the issues that were causing him such stress as well as getting him to realize he had experienced a panic attack.'

KEY POINTS

Stress is increased by a range of biological, social and psychological factors:

- Shift work disrupts bodily rhythms, affecting sleep and concentration.
- Crowding can make people more aggressive, less helpful and withdrawn, so they are less likely to seek help.
- Personality can influence susceptibility to the negative effects of stress; type A people and those who are less hardy are more likely to become ill when stressed.
- Locus of control is a measure of beliefs about the source of the reasons for and solutions to ill-health. Individuals with an internal locus of control may be advantaged in dealing with the effects of stress.

CONSEQUENCES OF STRESS
Effects of stressors on health

Clearly, stress has a detrimental effect on health via its impact on the endocrine and immune systems. In addition, some stressors have direct effects on health, such as damage from loud noise (above 150dB), which can rupture the eardrum, but permanent hearing loss can also arise through damage to the sensitive hair cells of the inner ear (which detect sound) at 90–120dB, such as experienced in loud working environments. In addition to the obvious effects of noise, it can also cause raised blood pressure and other effects associated with stress.

Another environmental stressor, pollution, has direct biological effects on health – lead can cause brain and liver damage, arsenic is a carcinogen, ozone aggravates respiratory problems, etc. In addition, pollution can have indirect psychological effects on well-being. Air pollution may prevent us from going out, and may increase the risk of aggression and reduce the likelihood of helping behaviour (Jones and Bogat, 1978; Cunningham, 1979). Furthermore, the stressful effects of major life events seem to be exacerbated by air pollution (Evans *et al.*, 1987).

Cardiovascular disorders

The effects of chronic stress include **hypertension** and atherosclerosis (build-up of fat deposits in blood vessels). Hypertension is a direct result of high levels of aldosterone and high levels of fat in the blood caused by elevated cortisol levels contribute to atherosclerosis. Both atherosclerosis and hypertension can cause serious problems in themselves but they also increase the probability of having a heart attack or stroke.

> **Hypertension**
> High blood pressure

Evans *et al.* (1995) found that children living close to a noisy airport had higher levels of adrenaline (epinephrine) and noradrenaline (norepinephrine) and higher blood pressure compared to those living further away. Job dissatisfaction exacerbates the effects of noise at work. Annoyance was related to both noise levels in the workplace and blood pressure and that this link was stronger in dissatisfied workers (Lercher *et al.*, 1993).

Haque *et al.* (2011) highlighted how stress may affect cardiovascular health in pre- and post-menopausal women differently. Cardiovascular disease is reported to be the number one killer of women in developed countries. It would appear that the usual protection of oestrogen fades in post-menopause and if a woman's lifestyle is still stressful, the risk of cardiovascular disease rises rapidly. Pre-menopause, oestrogen helps to prevent calcification, it widens blood vessels (called vasodilation) and prevents lipogenesis (conversion of sugars such as glucose into fatty acids). However, without these natural defences, women with stressful lifestyles and occupations may be much more susceptible to cardiovascular disease.

Gastrointestinal disorders

Stress is associated with a number of gastrointestinal disorders. The sensation of 'butterflies in the stomach' is not dangerous in itself but, if we experience it regularly, it is likely to interfere with our eating patterns. Stress also causes high levels of hydrochloric acid in the stomach. This is believed to contribute to the development of stomach and duodenal ulcers. However, there is now good evidence that stress is not the major cause of stomach ulcers – they are the result of bacterial infection (Macarthur *et al.*, 1995). Harris (1999) suggests that the symptoms of irritable bowel syndrome (which includes constipation and diarrhoea) are worsened by episodes of stress.

Effects of stressors on social behaviour

As noise can affect attention, arousal and stress, it is likely to have an effect on social interactions. It seems to make people unpleasant; they are more aggressive and less helpful. Page (1977) conducted a field experiment in which a pedestrian (a **confederate**) dropped a package near a construction site. Under different noise conditions created with a pneumatic drill, the incidence of passers-by stopping to help was recorded. Fewer passers-by helped in noisy conditions, especially when it was very loud.

> **Confederate**
> An individual in an experiment who appears to be a participant but is actually an assistant to the researcher

Such results arise because people attend to fewer social cues under conditions of sensory overload – participants in Matthews and Canon's 'noisy' condition may not have noticed the cast. Alternatively, the noise may affect mood, making people less inclined to help when in a noisy environment.

From the results of a study conducted by Yinon and Bizman (1980), mood seems to be less important than attention. Participants' mood was manipulated by giving them positive or negative feedback on a task they had performed. During the task, they were exposed to either loud or quiet noise. Finally, the participants were asked for help (by a confederate). Yinon and Bizman found that in the loud noise condition there was no difference between helping by participants who had received positive or negative feedback. As there was a difference in the low noise condition these results suggest that the effect of the loud noise overrides that of feedback, either distracting the participants from the negative feedback or justifying it. It seems that interference from a stressor such as noise is more important than mood in determining social behaviour. So, for health and social carers in a busy, noisy department, the environment may detract from their ability to assist patients effectively.

The environmental stressor of air pollution, in particular cigarette smoke, can affect social behaviour. In a shopping centre, people on public benches left more quickly if a smoker, rather than a non-smoker, joined them (Bleda and Bleda, 1978). Jones and Bogat (1978) found that volunteers would administer higher levels of aversive noise to another person if they were exposed to cigarette smoke. These responses could be due to a direct physiological response to chemicals in the smoke itself or to the annoyance it causes. Nonetheless, such findings support 'no smoking' policies.

Effects of stressors in health and social care work settings

Can stress affect health and social care professionals in their job? Occupational stress has recently been assessed in a study by Nabirye *et al.* (2011). They examined 333 nurses in Uganda and got them to complete questionnaires about occupational stress, job satisfaction and job performance. To qualify for the study, the participants had to be a qualified nurse, have been full-time for at least 6 months and working in a ward.

In terms of occupational stress, two main findings emerged:

1 Those working in public hospitals experienced significantly higher levels of occupational stress compared to those working in the private sector.

2 The nurses who had worked more than 20 years reported higher levels of occupational stress especially compared to those with 5 or less years.

It should also be noted that over two-thirds of the sample were 'ambivalent' about job satisfaction and that job satisfaction scores decreased with age. More research is needed to see if the occupational stress is *causing* reduction in job satisfaction.

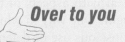

Over to you

Think about the above study and design a different study that might suggest that occupational stress *causes* lowered job satisfaction. Think about who you would ask and how you would run it.

Other recent research has examined the relationship between night work, occupational stress and cancer/cardiovascular risk factors in doctors. Belkić and Nedić (2012) surveyed a range of physicians and measured lifestyle choices, occupational stress and working patterns. They discovered that surgeons and anaesthesiologists both had the highest levels of occupational stress, which were mainly caused by longer hours and more night shift work. Also, only 12 per cent of the sample had a low lifestyle-related risk for cancer and cardiovascular disease (not a current smoker, BMI of less than 28, regular exercise and not consuming alcohol every day). Therefore, it would appear that occupational stress is affecting the health of senior health and social care professionals.

Having to deal with emergencies and/or longer term issues (like a natural disaster) can affect patients in health and social care settings. Edmondson *et al.* (2013) conducted a prospective study on the effects of Hurricane Katrina on survivors. Medical data were already available prior to the hurricane so the research team could directly examine the effects of the hurricane on patients who survived it. The survivors were contacted between 9 and 15 months after the hurricane for a telephone interview. Measures of health, post-traumatic stress disorder (PTSD) and depression were taken. These could be compared to level pre-Hurricane Katrina. Twenty-four per cent of the sample reported symptoms that showed PTSD (lifetime prevalence is around 8 per cent) and 48 per cent reported symptoms of depression. Over the follow-up time of three-and-a-half years, 158 participants died and a further 280 were hospitalized. Even though it was not statistically significant, those with PTSD symptoms had a higher figure for death and hospitalization.

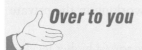

Over to you

Before reading the next section on coping with stress, how do you think we can help people who do suffer PTSD as a result of a catastrophe? Compare these with a fellow student. Are they the same? What differences do you see?

COPING WITH STRESS

Coping
An individual's cognitive and behavioural attempts to manage (limit, overcome or tolerate) internal and external demands in the physical and social environment that are judged to be challenging or beyond that individual's resources

Coping represents the ways in which we attempt to deal with aspects of the world that we find are beyond our normal means to fight. One way in which people attempt to cope with stress is through the unconscious use of defence mechanisms, as proposed by Sigmund Freud (1894). Individuals protect themselves from painful, frightening or guilty feelings that could cause stress, by unconsciously denying access to those thoughts or changing the way that they are interpreted. These mechanisms include:

- **Displacement** – the redirecting of emotions.
- **Regression** – the use of childlike strategies to comfort ourselves.
- **Repression** – the blocking of a memory so that it cannot be recalled.

If a stressful situation, such as an argument at home, makes an individual angry, they may use displacement and express their anger on other people, such as colleagues. Alternatively, they may become difficult – acting like a child – and use regression to avoid having to deal with the real issues. It is not uncommon in severe cases of stress, such as a traumatized road accident patient, to have no recollection of the stressful events themselves; this would be described as repression.

Stress management strategies

Sources of stress can be tackled from an external or internal perspective, that is, coping strategies can be either problem-focused, aiming to reduce the causes of stress; or emotion-focused, aiming to manage the negative effects on the individual. In any situation, a combination of these strategies may be employed.

Problem–focused strategies

Problem-focused strategies include discussing the situation with a professional, relying on one's own past experiences to tackle the issue and dealing with the situation one step at time.

Emotion–focused strategies

Emotion-focused strategies include keeping busy to take one's mind off the problem, preparing oneself for the worst, praying for strength and guidance, ignoring the situation in the belief that the problem will go away and bottling feelings up. Other strategies are listed in Table 7.3.

Table 7.3 Some examples of strategies that may be employed in response to environmental stressors (Note: These are not intended to represent the best ways to cope!)		
Source of stress	**Emotion-focused strategy**	**Problem-focused strategy**
Noisy children playing in the waiting area	Trying to remember that children need to play and it's good for them to be active (being objective)	Talking to a friend on the telephone about it in the evening (discussing the situation)
Smoke coming in the window from a bus stop below	Snapping at patients (taking anger out on others)	Closing the window (taking positive action)
You're on a night shift trying to work with the lights down but you can't concentrate because your desk lamp keeps flickering so you have to stop	Accepting that you'd probably make a better job of it tomorrow anyway (seeing positive side of situation)	Taking the opportunity to request a new bulb as well as gloves and bags that are also running out (considering alternative solutions)
You arrive on shift and the laundry room is a total mess	Eating or smoking more (trying to reduce tension)	Trying to find out who was responsible on the previous shift (investigating the issue)

How effective are the strategies?

It seems obvious that problem-focused strategies are better because they deal with the cause. However, it may be beyond the scope of the individual to effect change, so emotion-focused solutions may be essential to enable the individual to feel less stressed about the situation. For example, a patient could not reverse an accidental amputation, nor could a bereaved relative bring back their loved one.

Cultural factors also affect coping. Frydenberg *et al.* (2003) compared the way in which young people from different cultures dealt with their concerns. They found that, although all adolescents seemed to cope by working hard – perhaps to 'take their mind off the problem' – there were some differences. For example, Palestinian students focused more on social support, spiritual support and worrying than Australian and German students, who rated physical recreation highly among their coping strategies. Such differences suggest that it may be important to ensure that coping strategies made available to patients reflect cultural values.

In some situations emotion-focused strategies are detrimental; evidence suggests that long-term avoidance may be ineffective (Nolen-Hoeksema and Larson, 1999). Avoidance strategies may even be damaging. Epping-Jordan *et al.* (1994) found that, in patients using avoidance strategies, the progression of cancer was faster.

tɔɘ̱ʇɘЯ**Reflective activity**

Identify examples from your placement of patients (or staff) using emotion-focused and problem-focused coping strategies.

Coping strategies for health and social care settings?

Hunziker *et al.* (2013) conducted a study to test if a task-based coping strategy could alleviate stress during a simulated cardiopulmonary resuscitation. A total of 124 volunteer medical students from the University Hospital in Basel, Switzerland were split into two groups. The experimental group received a 10 minute presentation on how to cope with stress by asking themselves two key questions out loud when feeling stressed:

1 What is the patient's condition?
2 What immediate action is needed?

The control group did not receive any presentation. Prior to the 'test task' all students were made familiar with the resuscitation simulator. Participants in the experimental group reported significantly less stress and overload scores compared to the control group.

tɔɘ̱ʇɘЯ**Reflective activity**

Think about a stressful situation you have been in on a placement and assess whether asking questions like in the Hunziker study above would have helped you to make the situation clearer as to what you had to do.

Mindfulness-Based Stress Reduction (MBSR)

This is a relatively new approach to stress management. It incorporates meditation, yoga and mind-body exercises to teach people how to cope with stress caused by lifestyle and work. It involves rationalizing thoughts and feelings and teaching more holistic ways of coping with stress through breathing and meditation. But does it work?

In a recent review (Fjorback *et al.*, 2011), 11/21 studies showed a significant improvement in people undergoing MBSR although many studies failed to have a control group or a longer term follow-up. Also, Nyklíček *et al.* (2013) reported that community-dwelling people who reported high levels of stress showed larger decreases in blood pressure in an MBSR programme compared to a control group of no intervention. Furthermore, Wolever *et al.* (2012) noted that when an MBSR-based intervention was introduced in the workplace, there was reported better sleep quality and less perceived stress for those in this group compared to a control group. Bazarko *et al.* (2013) also reported success in a study that used MSBR on nurses. The 36 nurses who took part in the trial reported improvement in general health, decreased stress and decreased work burnout. The interesting thing to note here is that these improvements were still shown 4 months after the programme.

It would appear that health professionals have been interested in how MBSR may aid cancer patients. Recently there has been a review of MBSR specifically on breast cancer patients. Cramer *et al.* (2012) reviewed studies and conducted a meta-analysis on three studies (bringing a sample of 327 patients). MBSR appeared effective at decreasing depression and anxiety in women with breast cancer and they concluded, *'there is some evidence for the effectiveness of MBSR in improving psychological health in breast cancer patients, but more randomized controlled tests are needed to underpin results'* (p.343). However, a subsequent Romanian study (Degi and Szilagy, 2013) noted that in its sample, MBSR did *not* reduce negative emotions or improve quality of life but it did help reduce the isolation patients felt when trying to cope with breast cancer.

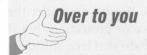

Over to you

There are occasions when, although taking action to reduce stress would be ideal, it is simply not possible – for example if you are a patient awaiting a diagnosis or a health and social care worker whose patience is frayed. What can be done to regain control? Rationalizing the situation can help. Imagine a situation in which you are due for an annual review meeting with your manager but there has been a crisis on the ward and you know you will miss the appointment. What cognitive strategies would you use?

- Informational control – find out as much as you can about the situation – how annoyed will your manager be? Will it affect the outcome of your appraisal?

- Decisional control – make a choice and stick to it – get on with it, pray, or try to get a message to your appraiser.

- Cognitive control – rationalize the situation – perhaps you could arrange to have the meeting rescheduled? – or recognize that, even if you had gone, you would have done badly as your mind would have been elsewhere.

- Retrospective control – reflect on the way you reacted, decide what you have gained – maybe that you should book important events outside your working hours or that you value patients more than meetings.

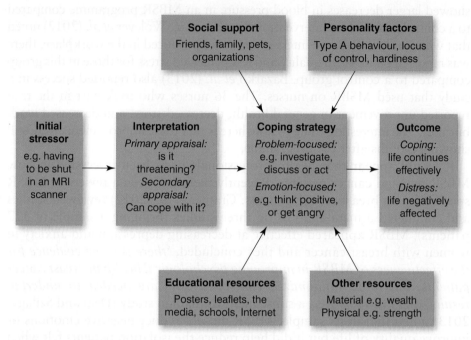

Figure 7.3   Coping with stress

RESOURCES TO HELP WITH STRESS MANAGEMENT

Different individuals, circumstances or situations may lead to the availability of differing resources to assist with coping, Figure 7.3. Wealth may offer the means to overcome many stressors (through avoidance or protection) but it may not provide a solution to inescapable sources of stress. Here, intrapersonal resources may be of greater significance. Wealth has been demonstrated to be linked to reduced stress but this does not apply to everyone (tending only to be important at the lower end of the socioeconomic scale, (Dohrenwend, 1973)). Neither is wealth a buffer against all sources of stress; it is not particularly important following bereavement, for example (Stroebe and Stroebe, 1987).

Social resources

People gain help, reassurance and assistance from their interactions with others (including their pets), which helps them to deal with stress; this is called social support. One way that people help to combat the stress of living in a time of political violence is to rely on support from others. How can an individual's social contacts provide support during stressful experiences? The kinds of support offered by social networks has been categorized in a number of different ways (e.g. Cohen and Wills, 1985; Stroebe and Stroebe, 1987). These are summarized by Stroebe (2000) in Table 7.4.

Table 7.4 Resources for coping with stressors		
Type of resource	**Examples**	**Ways they might be employed**
Material	Wealth	Having more money might enable people to pay for private health insurance and avoid stressful delays
Educational	Published research (including posters, leaflets and media information) schools, Internet	Knowing how to find recipes for meals with low salt or fat content
Physical	Strength, health	Individuals without asthma may be more tolerant of some air pollutants
Intrapersonal	Skills, abilities and personality characteristics such as determination and self-esteem	One individual might be better able to work effectively on a crowded ward than another
Social	Family, friends, pets, neighbours, community organizations	Being able to talk to the family dog about an impending operation may alleviate some of the fears about the procedure

- **emotional support** – providing empathy, care, love and trust.
- **instrumental support** – direct help such as caring for children or offering transport.
- **informational support** – providing routes to knowledge and understanding that will help individuals to cope with their problems.
- **appraisal support** – providing information that will specifically help the individual's self-evaluation, such as being able to compare oneself to another individual.

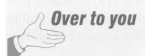 *Over to you*

Consider the following potential social resources that could relieve stress for someone enduring a personal crisis such as a diagnosis of a terminal disease. How would you categorize them using the Stroebe (2000) model?

Money, companionship, encouragement, leaflets about the problem, doing their washing, finding case studies of other people with similar difficulties, giving them web addresses for Internet support groups, offering compliments that boost their self-esteem, taking them to local groups dealing with their issues.

One source of social support for health professionals is other members of their team. Carter and West (1999) found that NHS employees who worked within a clearly defined team were less likely to suffer from stress, and they also reported greater job satisfaction and commitment than among those who did not work in a team. They suggest that teamwork helps people to cope by providing clear goals, an understanding of expectations and higher social support. Importantly, team members can provide a buffer against the negative effects of the working environment, such as poor communication and co-operation and a lack of resources and training.

Social support can be measured in two ways:

- Perceived support considers the respondent's description of individuals they could rely upon for assistance, such as who they could discuss an intimate problem with or ask for advice.

- Received support is the actual frequency with which an individual has gained specific supportive behaviours from others.

These two measures appear to be linked, but the relationship is not strong (e.g. Dunkel-Schetter and Bennett, 1990). This may be the consequence of the ways in which different individuals use others to assist them – talking to one person often or many people occasionally. For example, surprisingly perceived support may be a better predictor of health status than actual support.

Studying actual support is relatively simple; the inventory of socially supportive behaviours (Barrera et al., 1981) asks respondents about specific supportive behaviours in the domains of emotional, tangible, cognitive-informational and direct guidance support. An average is generated for each respondent based on the total number of occurrences of such assistance in the previous 4 weeks. Perceived support can also be assessed using questionnaires, such as the interpersonal support evaluation list (ISEL; Cohen et al., 1985). The ISEL measures four sources of social support: tangible, appraisal, self-esteem and belonging.

There is good evidence to show that social support is an important variable in health status. For example, Berkman and Syme (1979) found that those individuals with low social support had roughly twice the mortality risk of high scoring individuals over the 9 years following assessment of their initial health and social support.

Berkman and Syme used subjective self-report measures of health status. However, in a subsequent study, House et al. (1982) used more objective measures of health. These included testing blood pressure, cholesterol level and respiratory function, and electrocardiography. They, too, found that after a 10–12-year follow-up period, the mortality risk was approximately double for people with a low level of social support.

Buffering hypothesis

This model proposes that social support protects the individual from the negative effects of stress, either by enabling socially supported individuals to appraise stressful situations differently or by enhancing their ability to cope with the stressor. For example, an effective social network may enable stressed individuals to appraise a physical disability in a less damaging way because they recognize that they have people who can offer them advice or financial assistance. Alternatively, individuals may deal with the disability better precisely because they have those sources of advice and assistance.

If the buffering hypothesis is correct, the effects of social support should only be seen when stress levels are high. This is rather like the consequence of inoculation against a disease; if you have an influenza injection you appear identical to someone who has not, until you are exposed to the flu virus – under these conditions, your vaccination protects you against the disease. Likewise, buffering would only come into effect when the stressed individual's own resources were insufficient. DeLongis *et al.* (1988) investigated the stress levels, self-esteem and health of 75 married couples. Those individuals in unsupportive relationships (i.e. low social support) with low self-esteem became more ill in stressful situations than did individuals in supportive relationships with high self-esteem.

The main effect hypothesis

An alternative to the buffering hypothesis, this model suggests that an absence of social support is in itself stressful and is the cause (rather than the consequence) of ill-health. Social encounters are often positive and rewarding experiences and community membership can provide us with a sense of belonging and raise our self-esteem. This would imply that social support would be important to health regardless of stress levels. Hence the main effect hypothesis would predict that people with stronger social networks should be healthier regardless of the stressors they encounter.

The main effect hypothesis is also supported by empirical evidence. Lin *et al.* (1979) investigated the relationship between social support and psychiatric symptoms. They used information about participants' interactions with friends and neighbours and their community involvement as measures of social support. They found that those individuals with higher levels of social contact had lower levels of psychiatric symptoms irrespective of their stress levels. This supports the main effect hypothesis. However, as this was a **correlational** study, it is possible that individuals with psychiatric symptoms found it more difficult to establish or maintain social contacts; causality between the two variables cannot be determined.

It would appear that, when social support is measured as the absolute number of different social contacts that could be relied upon, results appear to be consistent with the main effect hypothesis. However, if social support is assessed functionally, in terms of the roles that social contacts can play in offering support, the buffering hypothesis is supported (Bishop, 1994).

Correlation
A relationship between two variables in which a change in one variable is associated with (but cannot be said to cause) a change in the other

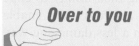

Over to you

Social support may help people to cope with a critical experience such as being an injured survivor of a traumatic event like a rail crash. Consider the two explanations for the beneficial effect of social support and decide which would suggest that people with high social support would benefit more in this situation than when exposed to day-to-day hassles.

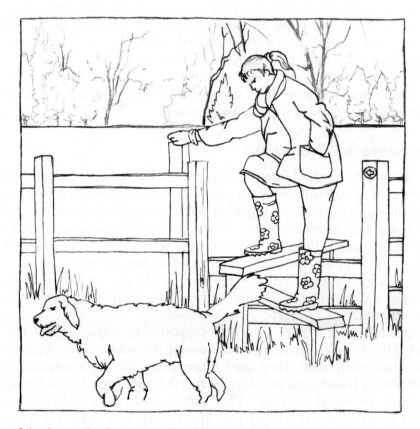

Going for a walk relieves stress. What helps you relax?

Educational resources

One way that the effects of stress on health can be mediated is through information, as knowledge underlies our health beliefs and attitudes, so is important (although not exclusively so) to the development of health behaviours. One of the roles of educational resources is therefore to provide knowledge and understanding about the health behaviour of individuals under stress and to suggest strategies they may employ to minimize and cope with stressors and reduce the associated health risks. Chapter 2 describes theories that explain how our health behaviours are controlled and discusses health education in detail.

Educating people to the risks of stress enables them to make informed decisions about combating the effects of stress on their health. In order to do this they must be aware both of the causes of stress that they are experiencing and the possible courses of action they can take to reduce the stressors or minimize their effects. Such information would provide the basis for judgements of perceived vulnerability to stress and seriousness of its effects, perceived barriers to taking action against stress and benefits of doing so. These components form the basis of health belief model.

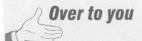

Over to you

If you have already studied the concepts in Chapter 5, you might like to use them to consider how you would plan a strategy for helping to reduce stress – *before* reading on.

The Mental Health Foundation, the Health Education Board for Scotland and the Royal College of Psychiatrists, among many others, provide educational information about stress. Broadly, this information covers:

- explaining what stress is
- the effects or symptoms of stress
- why being stressed is a problem
- the causes of stress
- potential ways to deal with stress.

Explaining about stress

One factor that affects an individual's ability to cope with stress is his or her understanding of the condition or situation. Educational information about stress can help people to feel that they can overcome their condition as it offers a means to gain control. According to both the theory of planned behaviour and self-empowerment approaches, an individual's perceived behavioural control or self-efficacy is important in following through health behaviours. The role of control is also important in understanding why some individuals become more stressed than others, for instance in locus of control theory.

Symptoms of stress

Informing people about the effects or symptoms of stress has two benefits. Those people who are aware that they are suffering from stress may be reassured that the symptoms they are experiencing are 'normal' (i.e. characteristic of stress) and shared by others. In addition, individuals who are suffering from stress but are unaware of their condition would benefit from information to identify the problem. They may have feared that their symptoms were due to some other condition about which they may have worried unduly. In both cases information may allow the individual to take action to protect themselves from stressors in order to avoid their symptoms. According to the health belief model, knowledge about symptoms that an individual was already suffering with would indicate to them the extent of their vulnerability and hence might encourage them to take steps to protect themselves.

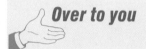

Over to you

Many different symptoms of stress are described in this chapter; how can they be accounted for?

How might a stressed person recognize their vulnerability to stress after reading information about stress?

Why stress matters

Modern society is competitive and success is valued highly compared to community-driven ideals. As a consequence, we may believe that stress is an inevitable part of people's lives so may be reluctant to act in response to rising stressors. This inertia can result in chronic stress responses that can be very harmful. Educating people about the risks of stress enables them to take action against the effects of the stressors on their health, so educational strategies aiming to tackle stress need to challenge the role played by society in passively accepting stress as a consequence of modern life.

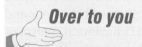

Over to you

With adequate support, people suffering from stress recover when the stressors are reduced. What advantages might a stressed individual perceive in changing their behaviour?

How could you challenge the subjective norm that we should expect modern life to be stressful?

Causes of stress

In order for people to improve their health behaviours they need to be aware of the causes of stress that they are experiencing. This will enable them to avoid or reduce these stressors so preventing themselves from becoming chronically stressed. Again, the health belief model would suggest that such advice should, in order to be most effective, indicate the benefits to the individual in changing their health behaviours.

Potential ways to deal with stress

When people have sufficient understanding of their own stress and its causes they need to know how to take appropriate action. The final role of education about stress is to inform people about the possible courses of action they can take to reduce the stressors or minimize their effects. In order for individuals to benefit from such resources, once they know that they are available, they must feel able to access them. Stress education must aim to break down the barriers that exist to seeking help in these circumstances. This is important, as according to the health belief model, people will fail to change their health behaviours if the barriers they perceive are greater than the perceived benefits.

CONCLUSIONS

The bodily stress response is mediated by both neural and hormonal processes. The sympathetic adrenal medullary system responds quickly to immediate threats while the hypothalamic-pituitary-adrenocortical axis maintains a prolonged response to chronic stressors. This stress response is caused by a range of factors, both internal, such as our own thoughts or pain, and external, such as pressures of work or crowds. Biological factors such as the disruption of body rhythms, for example by shift work, and personality type may increase our susceptibility to the effects of stress. These factors can interact, compounding the effects on our ability to cope.

The effects of stress on the immune system are indirect. Although short-term stress may enhance our immune response, in the long term stress induces immunosuppression. As a consequence, chronic stress increases the risk of succumbing to infections and cancer. Psychoneuro-immunology investigates the link between stress, immunity and disease. In addition to this direct effect there are other consequences of stress, on health performance and social behaviour. Stressed people may suffer cardiovascular and gastrointestinal disorders, have poorer concentration and are more aggressive and less helpful.

People may use emotion- or problem-focused strategies to deal with stress, the latter being more effective but not always possible. Social support and educational resources can help people to resist the negative effects of stress.

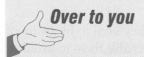

Over to you

Find some different sources of information on dealing with stress, you might try in your doctors' surgery, at a local counselling service and on the Internet. Critically consider the advice given in the documents. Can you decide what strategies are being recommended? Justify the advice offered on the basis of the empirical evidence available to support each strategy.

RAPID RECAP

1 Outline a biological mechanism involved in stress.

2 Outline the transactional model of stress (Lazarus).

3 How can stressors affect you in the workplace?

4 Describe and evaluate one way we could cope with stress.

If you have difficulty with any of the questions, read through the section again to refresh your understanding before moving on.

KEY REFERENCES

Other references are listed on the supporting website.

Baum, A. and Valins, S. (1977) *Architecture and social behavior: Psychological studies of social density.* NJ Lawrence Erlbaum, Hillsdale, NJ.

Holmes, T.H. and Rahe, R.H. (1967) The social readjustment rating scale. *Journal of Psychosomatic Research*, **11**: 213–218.

CHAPTER 8

PAIN

LEARNING OBJECTIVES

By the end of this chapter you should be able to:

- describe pain in terms of its physiology and psychology

- describe and evaluate the ways that pain can be measured

- understand the factors affecting the perception of pain

- describe and evaluate explanations of theories of pain

- describe methods of pain relief and relate them to theories of pain.

The Nursing & Midwifery Council (2010) say that the '...workforce of nurses numbers over half a million, so what they do and how they do it has enormous influence on the alleviation of pain and distress...' (p. 1). So, an important role for health and social care professionals is to limit the suffering of their patients. In Western medicine, this is typically achieved using drugs. However, there are other solutions to patient pain and patients themselves have a range of strategies that help them to cope with the pain they experience. An understanding of the nature of pain, factors that affect the patient's perception and the resulting pain behaviours will give you an insight into patients' experiences. A consideration of the ways in which pain can be managed, both professionally and by patients themselves, will enable you to support patients more effectively.

THE NATURE OF PAIN

Pain is one of the most intense feelings we can experience, yet our memory for it is oddly poor. We do, however, have a rich variety of words to describe the various forms of pain we can feel. There are dull aches, stabbing pains, 'hot' and 'cold' pains and pains that are mild, excruciating, nagging, burning, crushing, sickening or twisting. Clearly it is important, but what is it? It is related to physical harm – banging your head hurts – but it seems to be a lot more than just a simple reaction to injury. Pain has been defined as 'an unpleasant sensory and emotional experience associated with actual or potential tissue damage, or as described in terms of such damage' (International Association for the Study of Pain Subcommittee on Taxonomy, 1979). In other words, pain hurts, physically and mentally, and arises when the body has been damaged or feels as though it has.

This definition identifies several aspects of the experience. Pain is:

- A **neural** message that reaches the brain, so that we are aware of it.
- Unpleasant, so it acts as a warning about or indication of damage to the body (although not all pain is 'useful', as some is unrelated to damage).
- Related to our senses, as it can be felt through any of them yet is different in nature from our ordinary sensations.
- Affected by psychological as well as physical factors – a stimulus that is painful in one context may not be in another.

This definition recognizes the role that psychological factors can play in altering the way we experience pain, even if they are not the cause. Nevertheless, the definition assumes that all pain is of peripheral origin, although evidence does exist that some pain is psychogenic, i.e. it originates within the brain itself, see Figure 8.1.

We can consider different 'dimensions' of pain. Four have been identified by Loeser (1989). These are:

- **nociception** – the detection of tissue damage (a sensory experience).
- **pain** – the perception of that damage (interpreting the sensation).
- **suffering** – the extent of distress (how much it hurts).
- **pain behaviour** – the action taken that indicates tissue damage (both effective, such as putting a burn in cold water, or ineffective, such as swearing).

Neural
Relating to neurones or the nervous system

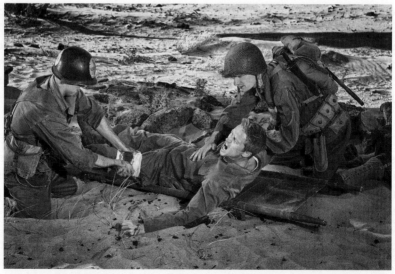

Figure 8.1   Our experience of pain depends on psychological factors. Beecher (1956) reported that soldiers who were badly injured in battle suffered considerably less pain than civilians with similar injuries. Think about how much your toe seems to hurt if you stub it when alone in the house compared to when you are with someone you want to impress with your bravery!

This classification is useful because it allows us to recognize that aspects of the pain experience may be independent. We may have extensive tissue damage but not suffer, for instance if we are anaesthetized. In other situations we may have relatively less damage but experience more pain. It is even possible to experience intense pain that appears to originate from a limb that has been amputated, as for some patients with a 'phantom limb'. It is therefore important for health and social care professionals to recognize that patients may differ considerably in their experience of pain even when they have apparently identical physical conditions.

Melzack (1973) suggested that several factors might influence our perception of pain. These include attention, suggestion (priming that suggests we will or will not experience pain), anxiety, depression, learning (e.g. being conditioned to anticipate pain) and cultural expectations. This range of factors also suggests that there may be at least two aspects to the pain experience, since it has both a sensory component (e.g. where the pain is or what it feels like) and a psychological one (through which these influences could act).

Priming
Preparing the body to expect a specific stimulus

KEY POINT

Pain:

- is caused by our interpretation of tissue damage, detected neurally
- is unpleasant, causing suffering, which may be increased or decreased by psychological factors
- results in pain-related behaviours.

Reflective activity

If you have had the opportunity to observe or interact with more than one patient with the same physical damage (such as postoperative pain from identical surgery) consider what factors, other than the physical sensation from the site itself, could cause differences in the experience of pain for those individuals. Think also about the extent to which these patients have differed in their requests for analgesia.

TECHNIQUES FOR MEASURING PAIN

When researchers explore the various aspects of pain, and clinicians medicate, they need to be able to measure pain. This can be done in different ways, focusing on the physical, or the emotional, component.

The self-report is a technique used both in research and in the context of health and social care, where nurses must assess patients' pain in order to collect information needed to make clinical judgements about the need for treatment. The individual describes his or her own experience, often using a chart to record the site and intensity of pain. Any pain relief administered may also be recorded here.

An alternative way to assess pain that has been used in clinical settings is based on psychophysics. This is a branch of psychology, which applies techniques from physics to assess our experiences, and makes use of a measurement called a threshold (the smallest stimulus that can be detected), such as the faintest noise we can hear. For staff working with patients, two pain intensities are useful: the pain threshold (the point at which the patient perceives pain) and the pain tolerance point (the level at which the patient resists pain, e.g. by restricting the movement of a painful joint). The difference between these two levels provides a third measure, the pain sensitivity range. This, combined with the drug request point (the pain intensity at which the patient asks for pain relief) can help to guide clinical decisions.

Techniques used in research

This section will consider the usefulness of different measures of pain. In order to assess tools that measure pain, validity, reliability and the extent to which the measure is subjective or objective are useful.

A measure of pain which is **reliable** would record similar pain levels each time it was used in a similar situation, i.e. a patient would give the same answers if tested twice. A **valid** measure of pain does not relate to some other factor, such as fear or embarrassment. If two independent measures of a patient's pain, such as their response to a direct question from a doctor and the observations a nurse makes, report similar pain levels they are considered to be valid. A subjective measure of pain is one taken from the patient's perspective whereas an objective one is independent, for example a physiological measure, such as pulse rate.

Self-reports and questionnaires

Self-reports using open-ended descriptions, include pain diaries, whereas more structured questionnaires are less subjective, so are more likely to be valid or reliable.

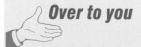

Over to you

Before reading any further, try recording in your own words a description of a recent bout of pain you have experienced. It could be backache, hitting your head or having a serious injury. Include information about the onset, intensity, duration and nature of the pain, as well as any impairment it led to and the actions you took (if any) to control it.

As you will have found if you have tried the activity above, describing your own pain is difficult, even when guided by prompts. If you compared your responses to other peoples', you may have discovered local or cultural variations in the way pain is described. When people are asked to self-report their pain they are generally given more directive questions. These may include:

- **Rating scales** – for example to measure the intensity of pain; these may ask for a score (such as 1–5, 1 being the most intense), a mark on a line (e.g. from 'no pain' to 'unbearable pain') on which the distance along the line is measured, or may have descriptors (such as 'pain free', 'moderate pain', 'as severe as any pain experienced').
- **Diagrams of the body** – to allow the individual to identify the apparent source of the pain even if they cannot describe its location.
- **Behavioural measures** – to assess the impact of pain on the individual's functioning, e.g. asking whether they can walk or climb stairs.
- **Forced choice items** – such as lists of words that describe types of pain.

The first three of these allow the researcher to measure the *intensity* and whereabouts of the pain but only the last offers an indication of the *type* of pain that is being experienced.

The most extensively used measure is the McGill Pain Questionnaire (Melzack, 1983). It uses diagrams and forced-choice items, e.g. closed questions where the patient chooses one descriptor of their pain, although it also allows for an open response. It aims to assess three key facets of pain:

- **Evaluative** – is a cognitive judgement about the intrusiveness of the pain (e.g. troublesome, intense, unbearable).
- **Sensory** – is a description of the nature of the pain (e.g. quivering, throbbing, pounding).
- **Affective** – is the emotional component of the pain (e.g. punishing, gruelling).

The McGill Pain Questionnaire (Figure 8.2) is both valid and reliable (Karoly, 1985), but it is not infallible. It does not distinguish well between types of pain and is limited by the different, and subjective, way in which we use language – people may be unable to find a word that satisfactorily describes their particular pain or may want to choose two words from one category.

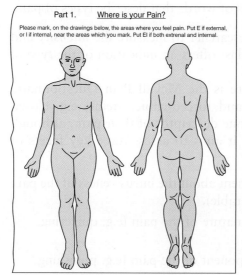

Mc Gill-Melzack
PAIN QUESTIONNAIRE

Patient's name _____   Age _____
File No. _____   Date _____
Clinical category (e.g. cardiac, neurological, etc.);

Diagnosis: _____

Analgesic (if already administered):
1. Type _____
2. Dosage _____
3. Time given in relation to this test _____
Patient's intelligence: circle number that represents best estimate

1 (low)   2   3   4   5 high
****

This questionnaire has been designed to tell us more about your pain. Four major questions we ask are:
1. Where is your pain?
2. What does it feel like?
3. How does it change with time?
4. How strong is it?
It is important that you tell us how your pain feels now. Please follow the instructions at the beginning of each part.

© R. Melzack, Oct. 1970

Part 2.   What Does Your Pain Feel Like?

Some of the words below describe your present pain. Circle ONLY those words that best describe it. Leave out any category that is not suitable. Use only a single word in each appropriate category–the one that applies best.

1	2	3	4
Flickering	Jumping	Pricking	Sharp
Quivering	Flashing	Boring	Cutting
Pulsing	Shooting	Drilling	Lacerating
Throbbing		Stabbing	
Beating		Lancinating	
Pounding			

5	6	7	8
Pinching	Tugging	Hot	Tingling
Pressing	Pulling	Burning	Itchy
Gnawing	Wrenching	Scolding	Smarting
Gramping		Searing	Stinging
Crushing			

9	10	11	12
Dull	Tender	Tiring	Sickening
Sore	Taut	Exhausting	Suffocating
Hurting	Rasping		
Aching	Splitting		
Heavy			

13	14	15	16
Fearful	Punishing	Wretched	Annoying
Frightful	Cruel	Blinding	Troublesome
Terrifying	Viscious		Miserable
	Killing		Intense
			Unbearable

17	18	19	20
Spreading	Tight	Cool	Nagging
Radiating	Numb	Cold	Nauseating
Penetrating	Drawing	Freezing	Agonizing
Piercing	Squeezing		Dreadful
	Tearing		Torturing

Part 1.   Where is your Pain?

Please mark, on the drawings below, the areas where you feel pain. Put E if external, or I if internal, near the areas which you mark. Put EI if both extrenal and internal.

Part 3.   How Does Your Pain Change With Time?

1. Which word or words world you use to describe the pattern of your pain?

1	2	3
Continuous	Rhythmic	Brief
Steady	Periodic	Momentary
Constant	Intermittent	Transient

2. What kind of things relieve your pain?

3. What kind of things increase your pain?

Part 4.   How Strong Is Your Pain?

People agree that the following 5 word represent pain in increasing intensity. They are:

1	2	3	4	5
Mild	Discomforting	Distressing	Horrible	Excruciating

To answer each question below, write the number of the most appropriate word in the space beside the question.

1. Which word describes your pain right now?   _____
2. Which word describes it at its worst?   _____
3. Which word describes it when it is least?   _____
4. Which word describes the worst toothache you ever had?   _____
5. Which word describes the worst headache you ever had?   _____
6. Which word describes the worst stomach-ache you ever had? _____

Figure 8.2   McGill Pain Questionnaire

Clearly, the second part of the McGill Pain Questionnaire (MGPQ) requires a good command of language, for example being able to distinguish between a 'smarting' pain and a 'stinging' one, which not all patients have. Visual analogue scales (Figure 8.3) are much less reliant on language so can be used by children and adults who cannot respond to spoken or written questions. For example, patients might be asked to indicate the pain level they are experiencing now, from the least imaginable to the worst imaginable, or to rate this for the past 24 hours. Such scales typically require a mark on a line between two extremes or to make a choice between graded images. Varni *et al.* (1987) developed a variation of the MGPQ that asks children to use different colours to indicate the intensity of pain in different parts of the body.

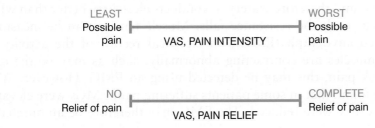

Figure 8.3   Visual Analogue Scales

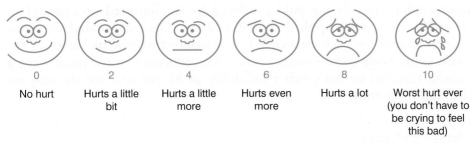

Figure 8.4   FACES pain rating scale (Wong-Baker, 2001)

Interviews

One important advantage of interviews over questionnaires is that, because the interviewer is listening to the patient's responses, he or she can alter the direction of questions if necessary. In a semi-structured interview the basic line of questioning is fixed but the interviewer can use discretion to collect useful information that might otherwise be missed. The product – a transcript of what was said – takes time and skill to use effectively.

Both self-reports (whether questionnaires or interviews) and observations can be unreliable. Patients may present aspects of their behaviour that they want to be acknowledged, for example, that they have difficulty moving or sitting if they want to take time off work. Alternatively, where closed questions are used, these may not allow patients to express themselves fully and symptoms may be overlooked. In observations, the observers may be biased (we tend to see what we expect to see), so a patient whom we believe to be recovering but who is struggling to conform to expectations may be judged to be in less pain than he or she is actually experiencing. As a result, we may choose to use a more objective measure – a physiological one.

Physiological measures

Pain is stressful, so some predictable stress-related changes could occur when we are in pain. These include changes in heart rate, sweating and muscle tension. Sweating can be assessed using galvanic skin resistance, a measure of the ability of the skin to conduct an electric current. When our skin is sweaty, and therefore watery, it conducts electricity better than when it is dry; as a result the resistance falls. Muscle tension can be measured with an electromyograph (EMG), an electrical record of the activity of muscles. If muscles are contracting abnormally, such as may be the case in lower back pain, this may be detected using an EMG. However, Wolf *et al.* (1982) found that in some patients suffering pain EMGs were elevated but in others they were reduced. The EMG may therefore be an unreliable indicator of pain.

Recent research has explored whether the subjective experience of pain can be detected with a brain scan. Brown *et al.* (2011) scanned participants brains before and during pain produced by standardized non-painful or painfully hot stimuli applied to the forearm. Once calibrated to detect painful stimuli for each participant, a computerized system based on the brain scans alone could detect whether the participant was experiencing a painful stimulus or not (with a reliability of 81 per cent for the easy-to-distinguish stimuli).

Observations

As someone other than the patient can make observations, they are more objective precisely because their source is not the sufferer. They may also be used when self-reports are judged to be unreliable, such as with children or people with cognitive deficits (e.g. stroke patients). The observer may look for:

- indicators of the patient's functioning, such as activities of daily living or attendance at work or school
- pain behaviours, including emotional responses such as crying or groaning and negative facial expressions and avoidance behaviours, such as muscle tension or limping
- requests for pain relief.

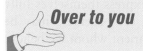 **Over to you**

The UAB Pain Behaviour Scale (Richards *et al.*, 1982) is a scale of ten target behaviours, which are rated for frequency by observers. It includes vocal complaints (verbal and non-verbal, such as groans and gasps), time spent in the day lying down because of pain, facial grimaces, posture, mobility, body language (e.g. rubbing site), support equipment (crutches, leaning on furniture, etc.), the ability to stay still and use of medication. If you have encountered a scale like this, consider how many of the items you were able to score well.

Professionals trained to observe pain behaviours use both 'covert' (hidden) but direct observations and indirect observations, e.g. using video. This widens the range of settings which can be investigated, e.g. to assess the impact of pain on work, recreation and family relations (Romano *et al.*, 1991). Videoing can be used for training to increase agreement between observer (Keefe and Block, 1982).

However, pain behaviours are reinforced, so may be performed more frequently than the patient's experience of pain would dictate. For example, a person may groan for attention, limp to avoid having to lift things for themselves or persist with the behaviour unconsciously because it elicits sympathy. Thus, observations may be flawed because they overestimate the actual experience of pain.

Health Care Professional

Clinical Psychologist

'Believe me, its not just in my head...'
'The first time I see patients they can be a little defensive, thinking they have been referred to me because their doctor thinks their pain doesn't have physical origins but instead is "all in their head". Many patients are angry because they have seen so many professionals and are still suffering pain. I ask them what they think is causing their pain and what it is like to live with their pain on a daily basis. I explain to them that my job is to understand what they think and feel about their pain so that ultimately I can suggest techniques they could learn to help them to effectively manage their pain. I work with the patient to develop a treatment plan that suits them and we modify it as needed over the course of treatment. This approach is successful in helping many patients to manage their pain.'

KEY POINT

Pain can be measured:

- for research or to guide clinical decisions
- using self-report tools such as questionnaires and interviews (e.g. the McGill Pain Questionnaire), observations and physiological measures (these differ in reliability and validity)
- with suitable tools for the situation, e.g. visual scales for children.

PSYCHOLOGICAL FACTORS AFFECTING THE PERCEPTION OF PAIN

We will now explore some of the psychological factors that modulate the perception of pain: they are, in their own right, important to patient care.

Emotional factors

Anxiety

A patient's anxiety can affect their experience of pain, and this can be self-reinforcing. For example, exposure to pain-related words makes migraine sufferers anxious (Jamner and Tursky, 1987) suggesting that they are sensitized to experience pain. This has been demonstrated experimentally. Unpleasant verbal suggestions cause a **nocebo effect** by producing anticipatory anxiety about impending pain, so the experience of that pain increases. Benedetti *et al.* (2007) have found that this anxiety triggers the activation of cholecystokinin (CCK), which, although a hormone, also acts as a neurotransmitter. In this role it facilitates pain transmission. Interestingly, CCK-antagonists have been found which block this effect and open up the possibility of new therapeutic strategies which could be important when pain has an anxiety component.

Fordyce and Steger (1979) suggested that there is a difference between the role that anxiety plays in the control of acute versus chronic pain and this appears to be related to the efficacy or otherwise of drugs (Figure 8.5). An anxious patient suffering from acute pain is likely to obtain effective relief with the use of painkillers (simply because analgesia is more successful in the treatment of acute pain). The success of the treatment reduces anxiety and this contributes further to the reduction of pain (see right panel below). However, in the case of chronic pain, the failure of treatment can exacerbate anxiety, leading to greater fear and a more intense perception of pain (see left panel). This could be explained by the cognitive effect of expectancy.

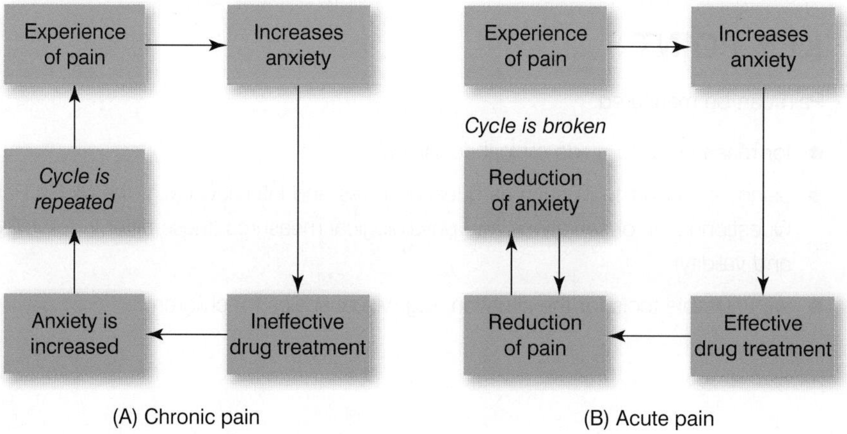

> **Nocebo effect**
> This phenomenon is the opposite of the placebo effect, so expecting a negative (i.e. unpleasant) outcome leads to the symptom worsening. Naturally occurring nocebo situations include the impact of an unwanted diagnosis on the patient or their distrust in therapy although it is ethically very difficult to test in artificial situations

Figure 8.5   The effect of anxiety on the experience of acute and chronic pain

Behavioural Factors

Learning plays a part in a patient's perception of pain. Individuals who have experienced pain before may have learned that pain, or pain relief, is associated with particular situations or behaviours. You may like to look back to Chapter 1 to remind yourself about the theories of learning.

Operant conditioning

In Chapter 2 we considered how learning theory could help us to understand ways to encourage people to acquire new health habits. The same explanation, of operant conditioning, can account for some variation in our experience of pain. Operant conditioning arises when an individual receives a reward (reinforcement) for performing a particular behaviour, with this resulting in them repeating that particular response. In the case of pain, people may receive reinforcement in the form of attention, sympathy or days off work as a result of exhibiting pain behaviours (such as groaning, resting or limping). However, as a consequence of the response they receive from others, their perception of the pain may actually increase (since these comments may serve to draw the individual's attention to their pain).

Classical conditioning

Another theory of learning is classical conditioning; this suggests that we acquire associations between stimuli when they occur together. If one stimulus spontaneously produces a response (such as a needle penetrating flesh producing pain and fear), one that is associated with it (such as the sight of a needle or being in a waiting room) may also begin to generate that response. As a consequence, people may learn that injections are painful, so become nervous in the waiting room or if they see a syringe.

Apart from the conditioned response, two other factors are at work here. One is expectation – the individual is anticipating pain. Therefore, classical conditioning can help to explain how experience may lead to increased perception of pain.

Conversely, the same process may explain the placebo effect. Since we tend to experience symptom reduction in association with taking medication, the response of pain relief is acquired to the stimulus of seeing and swallowing tablets. Since repeated exposure to this pairing of the drug as a stimulus and pain relief as a response results in classical conditioning, eventually the act of swallowing tablets that appear to be a drug will result in the same response. This arises in much the same way as a dog learns to salivate because it sees a tin of food – before it has even been opened.

Placebo
An inert (inactive) chemical or procedure that is administered to patients or experimental participants, who believe that it is an active treatment, and which produces an effect

Cognitive factors

Expectancy

Expectancy refers to the influence that our beliefs about possible outcomes have on our experience. If we have faith in a particular consequence or effect, then this is more likely to arise.

Expectancy and the placebo effect

Studies of the placebo effect typically show that when participants' beliefs are manipulated experimentally by giving them a drug reputed to be an analgesic, they experience more pain relief than control participants who received no treatment.

Several factors influence the effectiveness of placebos, including their size (bigger is better), form – capsules are seen to be more effective than tablets – and the number taken, and more dramatically, that subcutaneous placebos are more effective than oral ones and placebo (sham) surgery is most effective of all (Oken, 2008). At a psychological level, it appears that effects such as these are a consequence of the patient's expectations; the belief that a procedure will be effective plays some part in its success. De Craen *et al.* report that actual analgesics are equally effective regardless of colour but that whilst blue and green 'painkiller' placebos had some analgesic effects, red placebos were as effective as the actual drugs. Surprisingly, given the apparent power of the placebo effect, the producers of real drugs do colour their products accordingly. Khan *et al.* (2010) found no link between the perceived effects of different coloured drugs (e.g. that orange, yellow, and red pills are stimulating but green, blue, or purple ones are calming).

Both biological and psychological explanations are given for the placebo effect. The idea that it may be a psychological process is not necessarily in conflict with the physiological explanation, since expectations could initiate the central nervous system activity that triggers endorphin release.

Various sources of evidence suggest that expectations are important in the placebo effect. These include:

- Greater placebo efficacy if they appear to be genuine medication, for example if they look like drugs and are given to the patient in a medical setting.
- Greater placebo efficacy when they are administered by confident, high-status health and social care practitioners.
- The capacity of placebos to generate side-effects (commonly headaches and nausea) if these are expected by patients, in addition to alleviating symptoms.
- Similar effects of dosage, latency and strength of the placebo in comparison to actual medication.
- Placebo treatments with technological-sounding names are effective (e.g. 'subconscious reconditioning').

These findings all suggest that patients' prior knowledge about actual medication affects the outcome of a placebo trial – a foul-tasting tablet that requires a regular regime, prescribed with confidence in a medical context will be highly effective.

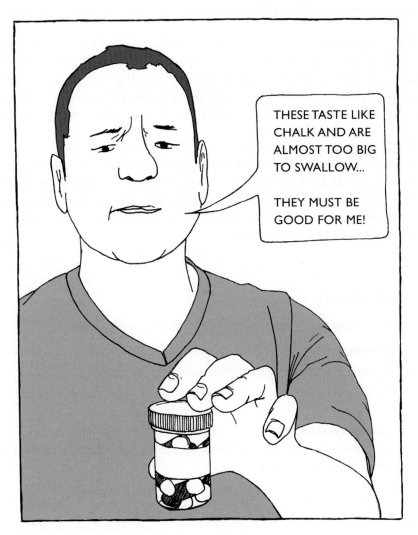

A foul-tasting tablet that requires a regular regime, prescribed with confidence in a medical context will be highly effective.

Gracely *et al.* (1985) investigated the effect of practitioner expectations on the effectiveness of a placebo. Patients having a wisdom tooth extracted were injected with either:

- aentanyl (an analgesic)
- naloxone (which reverses the effects of endogenous opiates)
- a placebo.

The patients were told that the injection might reduce or increase their pain or have no effect. There were two categories of patient: some could receive any of the injections, others only naloxone or the placebo. The practitioners knew whether patients were in the three- or two-option group but were unaware of their exact treatment. The doctors' expectations had an effect.

Only patients whom the practitioners believed could receive painkillers (i.e. those in the three-option group) experienced pain reduction. Since the patients did not know which group they were in, the only possible explanation is that practitioners' beliefs caused a placebo effect when there was a possibility of actual pain relief but that this effect did not occur when there was no chance of real analgesia.

Clearly patients' expectations are affected by many factors and can play a crucial role in their experience of symptoms. Incredibly, an investigation by Howick *et al.* (2013) comparing a range of different treatments and their placebo counterparts, has shown that placebos and real treatments often have a similar size and that placebos can play an important role, either alone or as part of a therapeutic regime.

KEY POINT

Placebo effects may be mediated by a combination of factors, including:

- **physiological factors** – the release of endogenous opioids such as endorphins
- **patient expectations** – belief in the treatment increases the efficacy of treatment
- **practitioner expectations** – expressed confidence in the treatment enhances the placebo effect
- **classical conditioning** – the patient's previous encounters with treatments that have resulted in symptom reduction will have built up an association between taking medication and pain relief.

Cognitive dissonance

Recall the sensation when you've bought something that maybe you shouldn't have – a new CD or a pair of shoes. You then engage in an internal process of justification – it might go along the lines of 'it's better quality/more unusual than this alternative'. The conflict that you feel is the consequence of cognitive dissonance. Festinger (1957) proposed the theory of cognitive dissonance to account for our tendency to make decisions that minimize our experience of tension because we need to:

- justify our behaviour
- perceive ourselves to be rational and in control.

So, according to Festinger, we debate the doubtful purchase, justifying it with thoughts like 'it was a bargain' to overcome our dilemma, allowing us to perceive the action to have been a rational one.

Cognitive dissonance and the placebo effect

Cognitive dissonance theory has been used to account for the placebo effect (Totman, 1976; 1987). It suggests that, precisely because we are prepared to make sacrifices – such as drinking revolting medicine or enduring the pain of an injection – there must be a corresponding benefit, namely an improvement in our condition. In fact, we make many 'investments' in our health, not least the payment of taxes or insurance to fund health and social care. In addition, we are likely to have spent time and effort seeing a doctor, as well as costs such as travelling or taking time off work.

This is only justifiable if we experience a gain; without any apparent benefit we would feel stupid or cheated. So we justify our behaviour by believing that the treatment works and thus avoid the feeling of dissonance created by perceiving ourselves to have been irrational. There is a 'choice', although not necessarily a conscious one. We could accept that there has been no change in our health but this requires us to accept that we have been duped – hence the dilemma.

However, neither in the case of research participants nor real patients can we be sure that cognitive dissonance is adequate as an explanation. Since it depends on unconscious mechanisms (the internal dilemma and a need to 'solve' it) we would need to independently demonstrate their existence to be certain. Nevertheless, this theory offers a plausible explanation for placebo effects, not just with regard to pain but also the relief of other symptoms using placebo treatments.

KEY POINTS

- Psychological factors affect the perception of pain.
- Anxiety worsens it, although in acute pain it can increase analgesic effectiveness.
- Operant conditioning can lead to behaviours to limit pain or to increase rewards such as sympathy.
- Classical conditioning can explain fear of potentially painful procedures and the placebo effect, through learned associations.
- Cognitive factors such as expectancy and cognitive dissonance are also possible explanations of the placebo effect.

THEORIES OF PAIN

Theories of pain attempt to explain how our perception of pain arises. An effective theory should be able to account not only for how pain originates but also how a range of factors, both physical and psychological, affect pain perception. In addition, it should be capable of explaining how pain-related phenomena such as phantom limb and the placebo effect occur. Finally, it should offer insight into the management of patient pain.

The specificity theory of pain

Early models, such as the specificity theory of pain (von Frey, 1895), suggested that pain signals are detected and conveyed along pathways of neurons dedicated to the function, i.e. that are specific to pain and are transmitted to a 'pain centre' in the brain. Furthermore, the volume of the information carried about a particular pain indicates its intensity.

This approach led to the belief that the experience of pain was an exclusively physical event (an automatic response to tissue damage) and research focused on finding specific pain receptors or nerves (clusters of neural fibres). Although some sensory receptors are limited to a single kind of stimulus, many are responsive to a range of stimuli, including pain. Take, for example, the photoreceptors in the eye that detect light; they additionally respond to pressure (a gentle movement of the eyeball through the eyelid of a closed eye will generate visual effects) and very bright light is painful. The range of triggers causing pain includes mechanical (e.g. crushing or distension), thermal and chemical stimuli. These are referred to as noxious stimuli and the process of detecting them is nociception. Pain receptors (therefore also called nociceptors) are bare nerve endings in tissues, such as skin, muscle, bone, joint capsules, ligaments, viscera and arteries. Intense mechanical stimuli are detected by nociceptors called high-threshold mechanoreceptors. A second type, the poly-modal nociceptors, detect noxious mechanical, thermal and chemical stimuli.

Nerve impulses are carried from the nociceptors to the spinal cord by two main types of specialized pain fibres. A-delta and C fibres. A-delta fibres are slightly wider in diameter and are myelinated and, as a consequence, send impulses slightly more quickly than the unmyelinated C fibres. The A-delta or 'fast' fibres receive signals from the high-threshold mechanoreceptors whilst C or 'slow' fibres take inputs from the poly-modal nociceptors. When the signals from these fibres, called 'first order neurons' reach the spinal cord, they synapse with 'second order neurons' that transmit signals about pain to the brain.

Nociceptors
Specialized nerve endings capable of detecting painful stimuli and relaying the message to the spinal cord.

However, whilst these pain-related fibres have been found (see Figure 8.6), Melzack (1993) observed that, if pain came only from specific pain receptors then the pain associated with phantom limbs should not exist By the same reasoning, referred pain should not – but it does. It should be possible to eliminate pain by severing the pain fibres – but it is not. Finally, the specificity theory cannot explain the variation in pain experienced with similar physical injuries (such as is demonstrated with soldiers, see Figure 8.1).

Referred pain

The **somatosensory cortex** maps out superficial bodily sensation, apportioning more space to areas with greater sensitivity. As a consequence, we can pinpoint 'external' or superficial pain very accurately. However, there is no equivalent 'map' of our internal organs, so we are relatively poor at judging the exact source of visceral pain. Moreover, visceral pains are sometimes misinterpreted as superficial ones – we feel a pain caused by an internal problem as if it were 'on the outside'. This effect can be very reliable and thus has diagnostic value – patients complaining of a pain in the shoulder may be referred for cardiac investigations, as heart pain is often experienced in this way, as *referred pain*. In other words, it is generated in a region that is relatively pain-insensitive but is manifested as pain in an area with a greater density of pain receptors.

The lack of evidence for the specificity theory and its failure to provide effective solutions for pain relief suggests that our experience of pain is a complex matter. In the course of this chapter we will consider two alternative theories that attempt to explain the phenomenon.

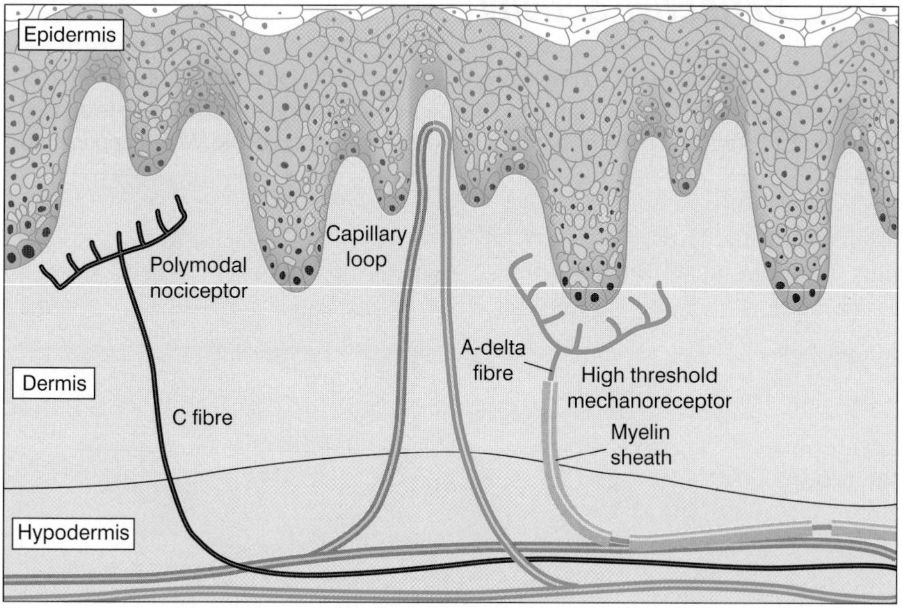

Visceral
Relating to internal organs

Figure 8.6   Two types of nerve fibres transmit pain signals from pain receptors to the brain.

The gate control theory of pain

The gate control theory of pain (Melzack and Wall, 1965; 1982) suggests that, although pain messages may originate as sensory signals, these go through several stages of processing during which psychological variables could influence pain perception. According to this theory, pain signals from the body are channelled through a 'gate' in the spinal cord. If this gate is open, the individual experiences pain, but this message can be modulated i.e. adjusted up or down, altering the pain perceived. The opening and closing of the gate, Melzack and Wall proposed, is governed by both physiological factors (physical signals from the body) and psychological ones (information from the brain such as memories about previous pain, attention to the pain or emotions such as fear). Figure 8.7 shows how the gate may act. The gate is the junction between the first and second order neurons. Because this is a synaptic connection, its behaviour can be modulated (affected) by the action of other neurons. Importantly, information from other, non-pain sensory neurons, such as those carrying information about touch, can act via an inhibitory neuron to close the gate. This would explain why patting or rubbing eases pain. Similarly, messages from the brain may also have an inhibitory effect and close the gate. This inhibition, in both cases, is achieved by endogenous opioids (see Figure 8.7 and next page). The process of sensitization acts in an opposing way, opening the gate and increasing activity in the second order neurons.

Reflective activity

Think about incidents where you have been in pain (perhaps you had twisted your ankle or developed a sore throat) then something happened to 'take your mind off it' – a telephone call, you hit your funny bone or became engrossed in a good book. What happened to the pain?

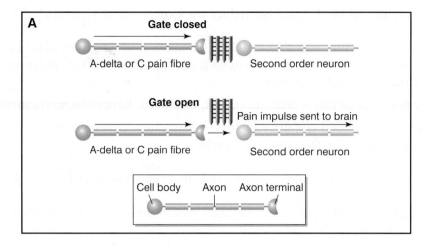

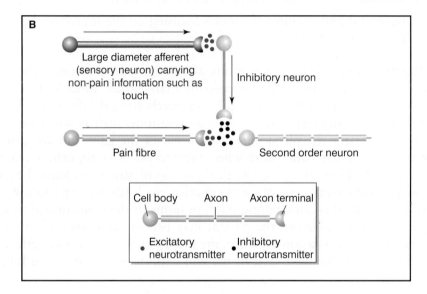

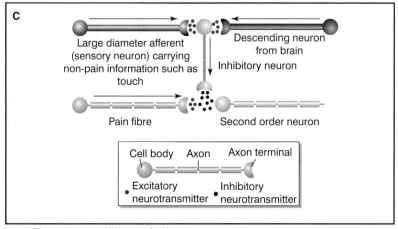

Figure 8.7   The gate control theory of pain

Factors that close the gate (so reduce the experience of pain) include:

- **physical factors** – analgesic drugs, stimulation of 'large' (A-beta) nerve fibres (e.g. by rubbing or scratching the skin), electrical stimulation of part of the midbrain area
- **emotional factors** – relaxation, rest, optimism, happiness, excitement
- **behavioural and cognitive factors** – distraction, concentration, knowledge that the pain will recede.

Factors that open the gate (so increase the experience of pain) include:

- **physical factors** – physical damage, stimulation of 'small' (A-delta) and C nerve fibres
- **emotional factors** – anxiety, pessimism, depression
- **behavioural and cognitive factors** – focusing on the source of the pain, expecting to suffer pain.

In terms of explaining observations about the nature of pain, the gate control theory is clearly more successful than earlier models as it can account for the role of both physical and psychological influences. It can also explain differing responses to painful situations, such as when we suck or rub a cut finger the physical sensation closes the gate, but we can be unaware that we are badly hurt when focused on rescuing others from a crashed vehicle. Here, the psychological process of attention closes the gate and so prevents pain perception. Conditioning leads to expectation; so when an individual is anticipating pain, in terms of the gate control theory the gate opens. In addition, the patient may become anxious and this will also open the gate. As a consequence, the theory indicates routes to effective pain relief and in the next section we will explore how some pain-killing drugs work.

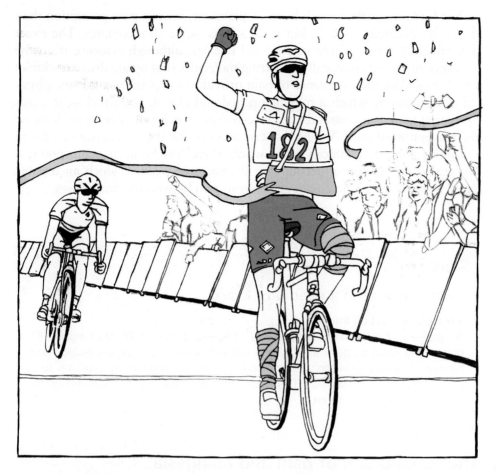

Signals about physical damage from an injury pass to the spinal cord and open the gate. However, psychological factors such as the lure of winning, being focused on the game and the cheering of onlookers counter this response and close the gate so the game goes on.

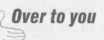 **Over to you**

Use gate control theory to explain each of the following experiences:

- Why an injection might hurt more if the patient has to wait.

- Why adults insist on a 'rub-it-better' approach to childhood injuries – and it seems to work!

- Why, in the absence of any difference in the physical nature of an injury, it hurts more when we are relaxing at home in the evening than during a busy day at work.

- Why a pain in the chest that you believed to be a heart attack might hurt more than an identical one you believed was indigestion.

- How having a massage could reduce a headache.

- Why sexual intercourse might decrease the experience of pain.

The GTC is clearly a much better explanation for our pain perception than the early specificity models, but it does have some shortcomings. The exact physiological nature of the gate is, still unclear, although evidence from the existence of opioids (naturally occurring molecules that opiate drugs resemble) which modulate the experience of pain provide an explanation for one physical mechanism by which it may be opened and closed. Nevertheless, it seems likely that there is a central (brain) mechanism, which can increase or decrease the perception of pain. Whilst this can account for the experience of pain in situations such as phantom limb, where there has been, at some point, a physical cause, it cannot account for instances of pain in which an organic cause is absent, i.e. where pain arises from purely psychological causes.

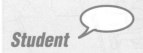

Student

Student nurse in a paediatric ward

Taking their mind off the pain
A 5 year-old girl was brought into my ward with infected eczema. The child was in a lot of pain and when a doctor tried to take a blood sample from her she recoiled and became extremely distressed. I distracted the child by drawing her attention to a cartoon that was on television. This helped to reduce her distress long enough for the blood sample to be taken.

The explanation of pain and analgesia

Endogenous opioids

Psychopharmacological substances
Chemical substances that affect the brain

Opiate drugs are those psychopharmacological substances that are extracted from the opium poppy or have a chemical structure similar to such compounds. The opiates include morphine, diamorphine hydrochloride, pethidine, codeine and many others; among them are some of the most powerful painkillers available. How do they work?

In order to understand the action of opiate drugs, you may wish to look back at the description of how neurons interact in Chapter 1. Opiates, in common with many classes of drugs, act by mimicking naturally occurring neurotransmitter molecules, fitting into the receptor sites for a particular class of neurotransmitter. The drugs, and often the receptor sites, were discovered before the naturally occurring molecules themselves. The natural molecules thus derive their name from the drug group.

Endogenous
Formed within, e.g. endogenous opioids are formed (naturally) within the body

In the case of opiate drugs, the receptor sites are intended to receive molecules from a group called the endogenous opioids (think 'internal opiates') that were discovered in the 1970s (Pert and Snyder, 1973). The endogenous opioids include the enkephalins and dynorphin – a molecule that is 200 times more effective than morphine at relieving pain. It seems that the opiate drugs function as analgesics because they mimic the body's own system for limiting pain. Pert has gone on to show that the endorphins, the molecules she had discovered, are also involved in functions known to relate to pain, such as emotions and the immune system (Pert *et al.*, 1998).

Research suggests that the role of naturally occurring opioids to suppress pain can be varied by a range of factors. Experiments investigating the effect of stress on pain perception in animals suggest that acute stress (such as in response to an electric shock) produces pain insensitivity, an effect called stress-induced analgesia. This suggests that psychological factors, such as stress, can trigger the release of endogenous opioids, thus reducing sensitivity to pain. Helmstetter and Bellgowan (1994) demonstrated stress-induced analgesia in rats in response to the stressor of noise. For one or two minutes after being exposed to a very loud noise, the rats were unresponsive to pain. They showed that this effect was the result of endogenous opiates by using naloxone, a drug that blocks the effect of both opiates and opioids by binding to their receptor sites. If the rats had been injected with naloxone prior to their exposure to the noise, no stress-induced analgesia occurred, demonstrating that stress-induced release of opioids must have been responsible for the initial pain-insensitivity of the rats.

Other factors that affect the release of endorphins include expectation, the timing and duration of painful stimuli, the individual's capacity to cope with the pain and their previous experience of pain (Sherman and Liebeskind, 1980). The factors responsible for opening or closing the gate in this list are similar to those in the gate control theory. This is further evidence that the opioid system is responsible for implementing gate control. Furthermore, Sherman and Liebeskind (1980) have suggested that non-drug pain control methods may achieve analgesia by stimulating the release of endorphins.

Acupuncture and endorphins

Acupuncture, used for centuries in China, claims to balance the two principles of nature, *yin* and *yang*, by correcting the 'lines of energy' (*qi*) believed to connect bodily structures. The technique uses long, thin needles inserted to differing depths at specific acupuncture points on the body, of which there are some 2000. The needles may be twirled, heated or electrically stimulated. Acupuncture has been traditionally used to treat a range of conditions such as headaches and arthritis. The practice continues, both in China and increasingly in other parts of the world, with considerable success.

Research suggests that acupuncture provides pain relief for some patients with a range of conditions. For instance, Coan *et al.* (1980) found that 83 per cent of a group of back-pain patients receiving immediate acupuncture treatment improved, as did 75 per cent of a delayed-treatment group. As with other treatments, it is important to distinguish the effects of the treatment from the effects of the patients' belief in the treatment, i.e. the placebo effect. To control for this, Vincent (1989) compared the effect of real

Endorphins
Opiate-like chemical substances naturally produced by the brain and pituitary gland to alleviate pain

acupuncture with a sham procedure and found that the effects of the real procedure on pain reduction were significantly greater, lasting more than a year post-treatment. Not all placebo studies have produced such promising results however (e.g. Dowson *et al.*, 1985).

Brown (1972) reported that, since the 1960s, up to 90 per cent of patients in China had undergone surgery with acupuncture, a procedure for which an electric current is passed between two or more needles. Acupuncture works for nearly everyone and the patient remains alert and interested (Melzack, 1973). Analgesia through acupuncture takes time to build up and is maintained by a continuous current. The effect wears off slowly, although it can be prevented altogether by applying a local anaesthetic to the acupuncture points. These points are very specific, suggesting that acupuncture may operate on a principle akin to referred pain, but in reverse.

Some studies, such as that of Hui *et al.* (2000), have used imaging techniques to demonstrate the location in the brain of the effects of acupuncture on people in pain. The findings suggests that acupuncture-induced analgesia is mediated by the activation of descending pain messages, i.e. signals that close the gate, according to the gate control theory, thus reducing pain perception. This view is further supported by evidence from Chao *et al.* (1999), who showed that naloxone blocks the effect of acupuncture on blood pressure. Since naloxone reverses the effect of endogenous opioids, this suggests that at least some of the effects of acupuncture must be mediated by endorphins.

RESEARCH IN BRIEF

Burns *et al.* (2007) Aromatherapy in childbirth: a pilot randomized controlled trial

Aims: To investigate the use of aromatherapy during labour as a care option and assess whether it could improve maternal and neonatal outcomes.

Procedure: The participants were 251 women having aromatherapy and 262 women having standard care during labour in a general maternity unit in Italy. Women in the aromatherapy group were randomly assigned to receive selected essential oils during labour, administered by specifically trained midwives. A range of intrapartum measures were used including operative delivery, spontaneous delivery, first- and second-stage augmentation, pharmacological pain relief, artificial rupture of membranes, episiotomy, labour length, neonatal well-being and transfer to neonatal intensive care unit (NICU).

Results: There were no significant differences for most outcomes, including caesarean section, spontaneous vaginal delivery and first- or second-stage. Significantly more babies born to control participants were transferred to NICU and pain perception was reduced in aromatherapy group for nulliparae but not the multiparae. The study, however, was underpowered.

Conclusion: As there were some significant differences but mainly non-significant ones, this suggest that the sample was too small to draw effective conclusions. However the study does demonstrate that randomized controlled trials can be used to explore complementary and alternative medical techniques such as aromatherapy.

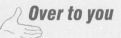

Over to you

Consider why the use of randomized controlled trials is so important, and why they present significant ethical issues.

In response to a painful stimulus, an area of the brain called the periaqueductal grey area is activated. This sends further messages through other brain areas and ultimately back down the spinal cord to the body. This route appears to modulate the pain signals, the inhibition resulting in a reduced perception of pain. If the periaqueductal grey area itself is electrically stimulated, a persistent and powerful analgesic effect is produced. Reynolds (1969) demonstrated that it was possible to perform surgery on laboratory animals using periaqueductal grey stimulation as the sole source of analgesia, and Basbaum and Fields (1984) have shown that direct injection of morphine into the periaqueductal grey produces significant pain relief even when it is used in minute quantities. This suggests that the periaqueductal grey is a key site at which opiates and opioids act. Further research has shown that the periaqueductal grey has a high density of opioid receptors and that it is stimulation of these that triggers the pain-relieving effect of the neural pathway leading down to the spinal cord.

Reflective activity

Think back to the ways in which patient pain, and that experienced by participants in pain research, would differ. In the light of gate control theory, how valid do you consider experimental studies of pain to be?

Endogenous opioids and the placebo effect

Placebos are inert, but have an effect. They are used in experiments in place of active drugs to control for any bias created by the experience of being treated. Analgesic effects and symptom relief have been demonstrated for placebos in conditions such as acne, allergies, asthma, cancer, diabetes, dementia, insomnia, multiple sclerosis and obesity (Haas *et al.*, 1959). For example, Beecher (1959) injected patients suffering from pain with either morphine or a placebo. Those receiving morphine demonstrated significantly greater pain relief, but the placebo was effective as an analgesic in 35 per cent of cases. In the alleviation of symptoms other than pain, however, placebo treatments do not appear to be effective (Hrobjartsson and Gotzche, 2001). So, how could the analgesic effect of placebos arise?

RESEARCH IN BRIEF

Levine *et al.* (1979) Placebo treatment for dental pain

Aim: To investigate whether the placebo effect is related to endogenous opioids.

Procedure: Three hours after the extraction of a tooth, dental patients were given a placebo injection. After a further hour, the patients received an injection of naloxone (which blocks the effects of natural opioids). Participants were given a baseline measure of sensitivity to pain and after each injection the participants rated their perception of pain on a standard scale.

Findings: The initial placebo injection reduced sensitivity to pain but the naloxone injection restored the participants' pain sensitivity.

Conclusion: The initial injection produced a placebo effect, however, this was abolished by the second injection suggesting that the placebo effect is mediated by the body's natural endorphins.

The findings of Levine *et al.* (1979) suggest that the placebo effect may be mediated through the endorphin system. However, as we will see in the following sections, many psychological factors are involved in the extent of a placebo response and this is one of the key criticisms of the gate control theory.

RESEARCH IN BRIEF

Engwall and Sorensen Duppils (2009) Music as a nursing intervention for postoperative pain.

Aim: To conduct a systematic review to investigate the effect of music on postoperative pain.

Procedure: Scientific articles about the effect of music interventions on postoperative pain in adult patients were sourced using online databases and included quantitative studies published from 1998 to 2007.

Results: Eighteen studies were found of which 15 showed a significant positive effect of music on postoperative pain. Four found lower use of analgesics for the intervention groups. The samples included patients undergoing various surgical procedures and the interventions were used at different times and included a range of music, usually chosen by the researchers.

Conclusion: Music can be a useful addition to standard pain relief techniques for the relief of postoperative pain.

The neuromatrix theory of pain

The last section illustrated a range of variables that can moderate a patient's experience of pain. These cannot be adequately explained by the gate control theory but can be incorporated within its more recent extension, the **neuromatrix theory** (NMT), which is discussed here.

The NMT of pain (Melzack, 1999) suggests that pain is a 'multidimensional experience', that is it is a complex, dynamic and active phenomenon. It is not only the product of the stimulation of nocioceptors, nor of the opening and closing of a pain gate in the spinal cord, but of the interactions of a sophisticated network. The key difference is the emphasis on a diverse architecture of dynamic central mechanisms rather than limited central interactions. This active system is called the 'neurosignature', a characteristic pattern of nerve impulses that is generated by the action of a diverse network of neurons in the brain, called the 'body-self neuromatrix'. Neurosignature patterns can be the product of sensory inputs, but can also arise independently. When an acute pain arises from a brief noxious stimulus, the sequence of events can be accounted for by nocioceptors and pain fibres. However, severe pain occurring in the absence of injury or pathology, such as in chronic pain syndromes, cannot be explained in this way but can be understood through the neuromatrix. The body-self neuromatrix generates particular output patterns in response to pain, for example after injury, pathology, or chronic stress, so the representation of that pain is distributed across a neural network in the brain rather than being a direct sensory product of that pathology. Because the neuromatrix is determined genetically but also modified by sensory experience, it can be affected by a range of influences, from simple somatic sensory input to complex representations in the brain.

The body-self neuromatrix is made up of many neural components, which interact in a cyclical way to produce their own neural output. This structure or 'synaptic architecture' is determined in part genetically and in part by sensory influences. The neural components include brain areas such as the sensory area, the limbic system and the thalamus, which are elements of the 'sentient neural hub' that synthesizes patterns to represent experiences. This is built up from three components:

- The sensory-discriminative (S) dimension includes the primary-level detection of physical damage.
- The affective-motivational (A) dimension includes the hormonal stress systems and the endogenous opioids.
- The evaluative-cognitive (E) dimension includes psychological aspects such as attention, anxiety and expectation and input from previous experience, both personal and cultural, in addition to one's personality.

The three dimensions combine, to various extents, to build the pain experience, that is, to create the neurosignature. This output of the neuromatrix is determined both by the inputs from different parts of the neuromatrix, spatial variables, and by when they occur, temporal variables and, in turn, dictates both the subjective experience of pain and its behavioural consequences.

Importantly, when the same patterns of signals are repeated within the neuromatrix, they generate a characteristic neurosignature, which can stand alone. It doesn't need to have the original sensory input to exist. This offers an explanation for the phantom limb phenomenon. The neuromatrix acts as a 'pattern generating mechanism' that, in limb amputation for example, may generate a pattern, high-level neural activity associated with the injury from severed nerve endings (Figure 8.8). This hyperactivity in central areas can then persist as a pattern of prolonged and abnormal levels of pain associated with the missing body part.

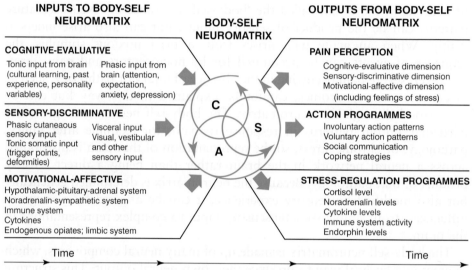

Figure 8.8   Factors that contribute to the patterns of activity generated by the body-self neauromatrix.

It is important to note that the NMT is not in conflict with the gate control theory, but represents an important elaboration of it. It provides a comprehensive explanation of phenomena such as phantom limb pain and expands the role that psychological factors play in our experience of pain.

KEY POINTS

- The specificity theory of pain suggested that specific pain neurons carried pain information directly to a pain centre in the brain, but this not well supported by evidence.

- The gate control theory of pain suggests that the intensity of pain signals arriving via the spinal cord can be controlled by the opening or closing of the 'gate', which can be done by physical and psychological factors. This can explain some aspects of pain perception that specificity theory cannot.

- The neuromatrix theory suggests that, beyond the stimulation of pain receptors and the action of the gate, pain perception depends on an interacting network of neurons which together generate a pattern of activation across the whole brain. This entire system detects and responds to physical pain and the psychological factors that affect the experience of pain.

COPING WITH PAIN

It is worth beginning this section with an observation from Krokosky and Reardon (1989) that health and social care professionals (including doctors and nurses) tend to underestimate the amount and duration of pain suffered by patients. This is problematic, since the role of health and social care professionals is to reduce suffering and it is generally accepted that it is easier to keep pain at bay than to allow it to become intense before attempting to gain control.

RESEARCH IN BRIEF

Puntillo *et al.* (2003) Accuracy of emergency nurses in assessment of patients' pain.

Aim: To investigate whether findings relating to the underestimation of pain in patients by health and social care professionals in inpatient situations also applies to nurses in an Emergency Department.

Procedure: Patients and nurses used a 0 to 10 numeric scale (NRS) to rate the patient's pain intensity in triage. The patient, the triage nurse initially completed this assessment (separately) and then again when the patient was being treated in the clinical area of the Emergency Department.

Results: Triage nurses gave patients a mean pain rating of 5.1, whereas the mean for patients' own pain ratings was 7.5. Later, in the clinical area, a similar pattern was found with nurses rating pain at 4.2 but the patients' own rating was 7.7.

Conclusion: There is significant underestimation of patient pain by nurses in both stages, which can have negative effects. Appropriate treatment may be withheld, so it is important to reduce the differences in pain intensity ratings, starting with careful evaluation and acceptance of the patient's self report of pain.

There are a number of different ways that pain can be controlled to the extent that a patient can cope. These include:

- Removing the patient's sensory capacity so that they feel nothing at all from the affected area, i.e. anaesthesia – the loss of sensation
- Removing the patient's capacity to feel pain in the affected area, although they may still be aware of a sensation, i.e. analgesia – the numbing of pain without loss of consciousness
- Altering the patient's perception of the sensation such that, although it is still painful, they are no longer concerned i.e. enabling them to cope by reducing their awareness
- Altering the patient's capacity to tolerate the pain so that, although it is still as painful, they are less debilitated by it i.e. enabling them to cope by increasing their resistance.

Some pain control strategies clearly use only one of the above processes; for example, a nerve block administered spinally prevents the detection of any sensation. Other strategies, however, employ a mixture of processes and it is not always possible to separate these.

So, the possible options open to patients and their health and social carers for coping with pain can be broadly categorized into physiological/physical methods and psychological strategies. Some examples include:

- physiological/physical control methods:

  - drugs
  - physical stimulation (e.g. counterstimulation, transcutaneous electrical nerve stimulation TENS)
  - surgical procedures

- psychological coping strategies:

  - relaxation
  - biofeedback
  - hypnosis.

> **Transcutaneous electrical nerve stimulation (TENS)**
> A system of electrical skin stimulation that is effective in reducing pain in some patients

Traditionally, patient pain has been treated medically, with predominantly physiological and physical methods. However, as our understanding has changed, for example the insight that gate control theory has given to the role of psychological factors in the patient's perception of pain, this narrow view of pain management has given way to a broader approach that encompasses psychological strategies too.

We will look briefly at the physiological and physical methods of pain control and then consider some of the psychological strategies (relaxation, hypnosis and biofeedback) in detail, but first we will consider individual differences between patients' own strategies for coping.

Pain, locus of control and coping strategies

In addition to offering specific therapeutic approaches to pain control, psychological approaches can provide health and social care professionals with an insight into the independent resources that individuals have for coping with their own pain. So, before we explore how pain might be managed, we will look at two aspects of the individual patient that affect the way in which they view and attempt to deal with problems including pain.

In Chapter 1 we described Rotter's (1966) locus of control (LoC), whether an individual perceives themselves, or some external force, to be responsible for the flow of their lives. The idea has been applied to pain by Manning and Wright (1983). Pain LoC assesses the level of self-determination versus external causation an individual perceives with respect to their experience of pain and affect how actively they engage in their own pain management.

Sengul *et al.* (2010) studied a group of patients with chronic lower back pain and found that, amongst other factors, high chance LoC scores were linked to higher disability level and pain severity, which had a negative impact on their quality of life.

A second patient characteristic is the idea of coping strategies, i.e. the extent to which the individual employs emotion- or problem-focused strategies for dealing with difficulties. Where there are useful steps the patient can take to deal with their own pain, problem-focused strategies are beneficial. For example, when adhering to appropriate schedules of exercise, rest or pain killers effectively limits pain, patients gain from being problem-focused. However, where there is little or nothing patients can do to minimize their suffering, as when an injured patient is awaiting surgery, emotion-focused strategies that allow them to ignore the problem or blame someone else will be more helpful.

Experimental evidence from Jackson *et al.* (1979) showed that participants exposed to inescapable pain (mild electric shocks), so they could only use emotion-focused strategies, experienced spontaneous endorphin-related pain relief. However, those exposed to escapable pain (i.e. they could take action to avoid the pain, employing a problem-focused strategy) did not. Affleck *et al.* (1992) investigated the effect of emotion-focused strategies (emotional support and distraction) on pain perception. They found them to be effective in reducing perceived pain when pain levels were low but they were ineffective for individuals with more intense pain.

Both of the above ideas are incorporated into the fear-avoidance model, which, in essence, suggests that, because individuals can experience pain sensations and behaviours separately, their perception of pain can become distorted. Importantly, it suggests that fear can enhance pain perception. As a consequence, it suggests that pain avoidance behaviours are counterproductive to recovery, so those individuals who confront pain are likely to make faster recoveries (Letham *et al.*, 1983). In line with this prediction, Klenerman *et al.* (1995) found that back pain patients who showed fear-avoidance recovered more slowly.

The management of acute and chronic pain

As we have seen elsewhere in the chapter, acute and chronic pain present different problems in terms of management. Acute pain, by definition, is short-lived (lasting less than 6 months). This alone may be important for a patient's coping. The knowledge that physical recovery will lead to pain reduction is an important psychological component, as is optimism arising from seeing physical signs of tissue healing (such as removal of a plaster cast or reduced scarring). These are likely to be absent for a patient suffering from chronic pain. Another important difference is the efficacy of painkillers. Both placebo and actual drugs tend to be effective in the control of acute pain but ineffective against chronic pain.

Furthermore, the experience of chronic pain often leads to a constellation of symptoms and behaviours that are self-fulfilling. For example, patients in chronic pain may:

- **be stressed** – this will exacerbate their pain
- **have limited social or recreational opportunities** – this will reduce their social support and increase their attention to the pain, increasing their perception of it
- **engage in pain behaviours**, such as complaining or avoidance, that may further limit social support, even from close relatives and partners
- **take a range of medications with little or no efficacy** – they may, however, have side-effects
- **suffer from depression**, which may increase their perception of pain and decrease the possibility of effective self-management of pain.

The differences outlined above suggest that strategies for the management of acute and chronic pain may differ considerably.

Physiological and physical methods of pain control

Analgesic medication

Morphine, a highly effective painkiller, is widely used in the control of acute pain, for example postoperatively and in the management of cancer pain. However, it has two significant disadvantages for patients who take it for a prolonged time: they may become dependent, and they may experience tolerance i.e. a greater dose will be required to achieve the same analgesic effect. As a consequence, other drugs may be used in preference to morphine. However, concerns about the risk of developing dependence (becoming addicted) are greatly exaggerated. The number of patients who develop dependence to prescription medication following surgery is very small indeed (Porter and Jick, 1980), whereas many patients with a legitimate need for analgesia are undermedicated or unmedicated as a consequence of such misplaced fears (Choiniere *et al.*, 1990). Weaver and Schnoll (2003) recommend the provision of guidelines to allow staff to use opioids confidently with patients with chronic pain, even including those with a history of addiction. Such advice can include using a medication contract, setting goals with the patient, giving appropriate amounts of pain medication, monitoring with drug screens and pill counts, and documenting the case carefully. So, to improve the use of opioid drugs for the first-line treatment of pain, NICE (2012) introduced new guidelines. The recommendations relate to:

- Communication – ask patients about their concerns and offer them access to frequent reviews of pain control and side-effects and as well as 24 hour access to advice.

- Starting treatment – for patients with advanced and progressive diseases, regular oral sustained-release or immediate-release drugs with rescue doses should be offered.

- first-line maintenance therapy – oral sustained-release morphine should be used as first-line maintenance therapy to patients with advanced and progressive disease and if pain remains uncontrolled a review of analgesic strategy should be conducted and, if necessary, specialist advice sought.

> **Patient-controlled analgesia (PCA)** A system of administering a pain-killing drug intravenously in which the patient has control over the frequency of doses (up to a predetermined limit)

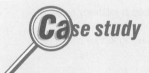

Case study

Eleanor – victim of undermedication

Eleanor, who was in hospital for routine abdominal surgery, was returned to her room after a prolonged period in the recovery room, during which it had proved difficult to get her postoperative pain under control. During the following night, Eleanor, who was still using **patient-controlled analgesia (PCA)** with diamorphine, called a nurse, as the pain was worsening. The nurse removed the intravenous line completely, believing Eleanor to have become addicted (less than 18 hours) and leaving her in considerable distress. The pain worsened during the following day and, although Eleanor had been seen by her consultant in the morning, he was recalled that afternoon. One glance at Eleanor's wound indicated that it had reopened and she would need to be readmitted for further surgery later that evening.

Reflective activity

- Was the removal of the intravenous line justified or appropriate?
- What effects, other than the significant increase in pain suffered by the patient, would have arisen from the removal of pain relief?

There are other, less addictive but also less powerful analgesics than the opiates. These include ibuprofen, paracetamol and aspirin. The exact mechanism of these analgesics is not, however, fully understood. A brief tabulation of analgesics and their properties is given in Table 8.1.

Table 8.1 Analgesics and their properties			
Drug group	**Examples**	**Mode of action**	**Disadvantages**
Opiates	Morphine, Diamorphine, Pethidine, Tramadol, Codeine	Mimic endogenous opioids	Risk of dependence and tolerance with long-term use; short-term effects of constipation, poor judgement
NSAID	Aspirin	Has several effects on the nervous system which contribute to its analgesic properties and acts as an anti-inflamatory.	Increases clotting time (problematic for patients with wounds); can cause gastric irritation; toxic in large quantities (causing liver and kidney damage)
Mild analgesic	Paracetamol	Reduces temperature but has little anti-inflammatory effect	Toxic in relatively small quantities (causing kidney damage)
Other NSAIDs	Ibuprofen, Diclofenac	Block synthesis of prostaglandins which are released at the site of damage or inflammation and sensitize pain-conducting neurones	Less effective on pain not associated with inflammation; can cause gastric irritation; toxic in large quantities (causing liver and kidney damage)

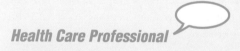

Health Care Professional

Consultant nurse

Pain management: an interprofessional approach
Pain management can involve a whole range of health and social care professionals, particularly pharmacists, doctors and specialist nurses. I had one patient on the ward with a cancerous mass and she was deteriorating quite quickly, and she was on oral morphine solution every 6 hours. We got the pain care specialist nurse to review her to see if having a syringe driver of diamorphine would be appropriate. Because as nurses we're there looking after patients all the time we have more indication of whether they're in pain and when to call in other health professionals. The registrar prescribed this, and she settled much better, and was not crying out when we tried to move her.

Physical stimulation as a control measure for pain

Counterstimulation is a pain control measure achieved by stimulating, or irritating, another part of the body. A possible explanation for the mechanism by which counterstimulation may work was discussed on in the context of the gate control theory.

Transcutaneous electrical nerve stimulation (TENS) is a system of electrical skin stimulation that is effective in reducing pain in some patients (Melzack and Wall, 1982). Electrical stimulation from the electrodes penetrates to a depth of about 4cm and the patient can control both the location of the electrodes and the frequency and strength of the electrical signals. When effective, relief following a session of TENS treatment can last for several hours and may be used to combat some instances of both acute and chronic pain.

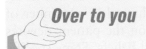
Over to you

If you have access to a department in which TENS is used, try to find out what it is used for and what benefit patients perceive with its use.

Psychological strategies for coping with pain

Acupuncture, discussed earlier, is sometimes regarded as a psychological technique for coping with pain. As research progresses, the physiological process by which the effects of acupuncture arise are becoming apparent. For example, Yang *et al.* (2012) used brain scanning to demonstrate that when acupuncture was used to reduce pain in migraine sufferers, there was a detectable change in activity in pain-related areas of the brain.

In this section, three strategies that are more clearly psychological in nature are discussed: relaxation, biofeedback and hypnosis. However, it is important to bear in mind that these strategies, like acupuncture and the placebo effect, must have underlying physiological mechanisms and they may ultimately be uncovered.

Cognitive behavioural therapy

One psychological approach to pain management is the use of cognitive-behavioural strategies. This approach recognizes the role of different sources of experience in pain perception and coping:

- **Thinking** – for example, what pain means to the individual 'I am in too much pain to continue with my job'.
- **Emotions** – how the individual feels about their pain, for example 'I'm frightened that it won't ever get easier to bear'.
- **Physiology** – the role of the nervous system, for instance impulses from a site of injury.
- **Behaviour** – for instance avoiding exercise because it hurts.

As its name implies, cognitive behavioural therapy (CBT) employs a range of strategies to tackle both cognitive issues, including thoughts and beliefs that lead the patient to focus on the pain, and behaviour – changing the way a patient responds to their experience of pain. Since explanations of pain, such as the neuromatrix theory, indicate the central role of the brain and therefore thinking in our experience of pain, it is logical that by altering the way a patient thinks about their situation will therefore influence their pain perception. This is not merely distraction, but an attempt to change some of the other cognitive and affective processes that influence pain perception.

A cognitive behavioural therapist aims to increase the individual's self-control over their pain and uses intrinsic (internal) sources of reinforcement to sustain these changes. This aim may be achieved in a number of different ways, for example by reducing the attention the patient devotes to the pain or to change pain related behaviours and beliefs. Some specific goals of CBT may include:

- **Overcoming demoralization** – feelings of helplessness can be restructured to allow individuals to see their pain as manageable.

- **Reducing counterproductive strategies** – patients may have learned maladaptive coping strategies, such as avoiding exercise, that actually worsen their pain; CBT teaches them to be aware of such feelings and behaviours.

- **Skills training** – adaptive strategies are taught so that the patient has alternative ways to cope; these may include refocusing attention away from the pain, thus reducing the distress experienced.

- **Increasing self-efficacy** – passive patients are taught to accept that they have control and competence.

- **Self-attribution** – patients may believe that success in treatment is attributable to others but that they are to blame if treatment fails; they are taught that they too can be responsible for positive outcomes.

- **Encourage future coping** – patients are taught ways to anticipate problems and develop their own strategies to cope with them, so that the effects of the intervention are lasting.

- **Belief in treatment efficacy** – patients with chronic pain whose treatments have been unsuccessful may believe that no treatments work; they are taught to believe that CBT will improve their condition.

CBT has been successful in reducing pain and improving coping. For example, Thomas *et al.* (1999) found that CBT not only reduced pain and distress in patients with sickle-cell disease but also helped their ability to cope. This effect was evident both immediately after the intervention and at 2 months post-treatment. More recent studies continue to show the same pattern, for example Hoffman *et al.* (2007) again found that CBT was effective with patients suffering from lower back pain. In a study looking at CBT for pain management in a wider range of conditions, Morely *et al.* (2008) used measures including patients' experience of pain, psychological distress (depression and anxiety), their self-efficacy, the extent to which it interfered with their daily lives and their ability to walk. Comparing pre- to post-treatment and follow-up they found significant improvement in many of these outcomes, with between one in three and one in seven (depending on the outcome measure used) gaining from CBT. However, between 1–2 per cent of patients deteriorated during treatment, so CBT is not effective in all situations.

As Morely *et al.*'s findings imply, the success of CBT may be the result of the intended changes in the patients' beliefs and self-efficacy. Dolce (1987) found that patients on a treatment programme who experienced reduced pain, but attributed this improvement to the therapist rather than to changes in their own skills, were less likely to continue to use the strategies they had learned and were more likely to relapse after the intervention. This indeed suggests that CBT may reduce patients' experience of pain by increasing self-efficacy.

Relaxation

Relaxation techniques were originally developed as a means to help clients with anxiety disorders such as phobias. Effective relaxation requires not only the reduction of tension in muscles but also a slowing of the breathing rate. During relaxation training initial deep breaths are followed by slower, deeper breaths than the client usually takes and they are more focused on the rhythm of their own breathing. Wolpe (1958) developed a technique known as systematic desensitization in which relaxed clients progressively lose their fear of previously phobia-inducing situations such as small spaces or snakes. Since this technique works primarily by reducing anxiety, and this is one of the key psychological factors in increasing a patient's experience of pain, it follows that anxiety-reduction should be efficacious in pain control. In addition, for those sources of pain that are directly related to or exacerbated by physical tension, relaxation should also reduce pain. For example, Baad-Hansen *et al.* (2013) found that relaxation was as effective as hypnosis in the reduction of idiopathic orofacial pain (although the techniques were different in their effectiveness with different patient groups). However, not all research demonstrates that relaxation is an effective treatment, for example, Abrahamsen *et al.* (2011) found a significant improvement with hypnosis for patients with painful temporomandibular disorders, no significant improvement was demonstrated using relaxation.

In common with other therapies, relaxation is likely to work better in combination with other techniques. Holroyd and Penzien (1990) found that relaxation was more effective than a placebo in the treatment of recurrent migraine headaches. However, this treatment was more effective still if combined with biofeedback (see next section).

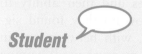

Student

Counselling student

The importance of relaxation in symptom control is illustrated by this student's experience ...

The one place where I saw the use of relaxation was in a group home for clients with learning disabilities. They had a 'relaxation therapy room' that had 'Austin Powers' psychedelic lights, throws and big, fluffy cushions. They used it for people with challenging behaviours, and when I was in there I felt that I could have floated away.

Biofeedback

Biofeedback is the use by patients of information about changes in their own condition to enhance their recovery. This feedback about biological status, such as temperature, blood pressure, heart rate or muscle tension, is provided to patients by giving them access to a standard physiological measure (such as skin temperature, blood pressure or heart rate monitors or electromyogram readings).

The process operates on a classical conditioning paradigm. This learning mechanism suggests that biofeedback occurs because the stimulus – such as a tilt-table used to produce a desired effect of reducing blood pressure – becomes associated with the new stimulus of thinking about the effect. After repeated pairings, classical conditioning results in the new stimulus, i.e. thinking about the effect, becoming capable of independently causing the desired response. This process has been used effectively to reduce pain in conditions such as Raynaud's disease (using feedback about skin temperature) and hypertension (using feedback about blood pressure). It is particularly useful as it allows patients to play a central role in their own symptom management and, furthermore, is effective with some chronic conditions.

Raynaud's disease
A condition in which blood supply, particularly to the digits, is over-sensitive to cold, causing circulation to the fingers and toes to fail

RESEARCH IN BRIEF

Shiri *et al.* (2013) A virtual reality system combined with biofeedback for treating paediatric chronic headache.

Aim: To explore the possibility of using biofeedback to achieve pain reduction in children suffering from chronic headache.

Procedure: A pilot study was conducted using ten children attending an outpatient paediatric neurology clinic. Each child had ten-session intervations of relaxation with biofeedback to learn to associate relaxation with a positive pain-free virtual image of themselves.

Results: Nine patients completed the all sessions. Their ratings of pain, daily functioning and quality of life improved significantly at 1 and at 3 months' post-treatment. Most reported subsequent use of the relaxation and imagery skills they had learned to relieve headache.

Conclusion: The combination of biofeedback and virtual reality, offers a possible intervention for paediatric use. To assess its use, randomized controlled studies using larger samples are needed.

However, despite the sound reasoning behind biofeedback, early evidence suggested that modification of the target process (such as lowering blood pressure) and reduction of pain were not necessarily related. For example, although some studies (e.g. Nakao *et al.*, 1997,) have found benefits to patients using biofeedback to reduce blood pressure, other have failed to find a lasting effect (e.g. McGrady, 1994). An area in which biofeedback works effectively is in changing posture to reduce pain. O'Sullivan *et al.* (2013) found that chronic low back pain could be reduced, at least in the short-term, using biofeedback to improve posture in seated patients. Giggins (2013) conducted a review of studies on biofeedback and found it to be effective for a range of conditions including hypertension, heart failure, asthma, fibromyalgia. According to this review, recent studies of biofeedback techniques, using virtual reality (see research now for an example), show it to be particularly effective, although further research is needed in this area. Other influences, such as relaxation or the placebo effect, may in fact be responsible for the beneficial changes observed in biofeedback.

Hypnosis

Franz Anton Mesmer (hence the term 'mesmerized') was the first documented practitioner of what is now called hypnosis. He aimed to use his skills therapeutically and believed that the effects he induced in people were a result of his own 'magnetism'. Although Mesmer is unlikely to have been magnetic, his clinical practice was demonstrably effective. More recently, techniques of relaxation, eye fixation – focusing on an object and verbal cues such as feeling heaviness in the eyelids – or a sensation of moving downwards are used to induce a state of hypnosis. Effectively administered to a susceptible person, these procedures lead to a condition of relaxed suggestibility that can have useful clinical effects. The hypnotized patient will respond to suggestions of imagery made by the therapist and these may be used to provide a context within which the awareness of pain is limited.

Both analgesia and anaesthesia are possible through hypnosis. A measure of analgesia may arise spontaneously during hypnosis; as the subject becomes absorbed in the imagery, their awareness of other sensations diminishes. This is comparable to not realizing we have gone numb from sitting still for hours reading a good book. A greater analgesic effect can be achieved by direct suggestion. This can result from suggested loss of sensation, e.g. as a 'glove' protecting the hand from pain, or by guiding the subject to feel separate from that part of the body. Other techniques use age progression or regression to take the client forwards or backwards in time to a pain-free age, and suggestions to 'forget' the pain (Yapko, 1995).

Health Care Professional

Clinical psychologist

Hypnosis, CBT and the treatment of pain

'A significant proportion of my caseload, consists of people who have problems with pain or a fear of potentially painful procedures. With these I use hypnosis as a context for teaching cognitive behavioural pain management strategies such as sensory transformation, detachment and imaginative inattention, as well as using direct analgesia suggestions.

Sometimes these can be very short interventions. On a number of occasions I have been asked by clients to help them to cope with a forthcoming surgical procedure – often this request has come the day before their operation. My usual method for this is the so-called "special place" technique, in which clients are taught in hypnosis to take themselves to a safe and relaxing place of their own choosing (warm, sunny beaches are very popular) where "nothing can bother them". After a single session of training they are then encouraged to practise this as their own self-hypnosis routine to reduce anxiety before the feared procedure and to cope with pain and discomfort during it.

Using a related approach, one young client with needle phobia was able to tolerate a routine immunization injection in front of her classmate. She learned in hypnosis to experience her arm as becoming detached from her body and to then use the same strategy in the real situation – leaving her arm with the nurse while the injection took place. For dental phobics it is often helpful to teach a hypnotized client how to make their hand feel numb (by imagining plunging it into snow for example) and to transfer that numbness by touching an appropriate part of their mouth, which they can then do later when in the dental chair. With chronic pain, such as that associated with fibromyalgia, some clients are able to reduce their painful experience in hypnosis by "turning down" an imaginary "dial" that controls their pain. One person who was suffering from a disabling chronic pain that had continued long after a whiplash injury had physically healed found she could divert her pain in self-hypnosis to the top of her head, where it would be released "like lava spurting out of a volcano". Similarly, a client with phantom limb pain, which she described like a "fizzling firework about to explode", was able to "douse" the pain by imagining pouring a jug of water over it. Both of these clients went on to apply the same technique for themselves in everyday situations using a rapid self-hypnosis procedure and found that their pain throughout the day was significantly reduced and sometimes eliminated.'

In addition to the treatment of fear of pain, hypnosis can also be used to reduce patients' experience of actual pain. Hypnosis is more effective than simple relaxation, for example, Abrahamsen *et al.* (2011) found that of patients with painful temporomandibular disorders those in the hypnosis group obtained relief but those in the control condition did not. Self-hypnosis has also been used effectively in pain control. Substantial pain relief can be achieved by direct hypnotic suggestion in 75 per cent of the population and more complete analgesia in about 20 per cent of hypnotic subjects (Montgomery *et al.*, 2000) so, although it can be used with most people, it is not a solution available to all patients. For those individuals for whom it is effective, however, it is sufficient for analgesia during surgery, dentistry and to relieve persistent pain, such as in cancer or burns patients.

As might be expected, directly suggested analgesia is more effective in high-susceptibility subjects than those who are less susceptible (Montgomery *et al.*, 2000). However, this relationship is not so evident when more broadly based hypnotic strategies are used. This suggests that some feature other than, or in addition to, direct suggestion is important in achieving the analgesia. These results may arise because low-susceptibility patients may be as good as high-susceptibility patients at employing more general pain-coping strategies explicitly offered by the hypnotist (such as relaxation and distraction). This view is supported by the observation that such strategies, including the use of suggestion, are often effective, without hypnosis, in producing analgesia (Spanos *et al.*, 1974).

There is, however, experimental evidence demonstrating the occurrence of specific suggestion-based changes associated with the perception of pain under hypnosis. Rainville *et al.* (1997) used positron-emission tomography (PET) scanning to track brain changes during hypnosis and its effect on experimentally induced pain. They found that activity in a particular area of the brain, the anterior cingulate gyrus, remained unchanged when hypnosis was induced but did change in relation to suggestions about the unpleasantness of pain.

The process by which hypnosis mediates pain relief is unclear. Apart from the effects of relaxation and distraction, a possible explanation is that hypnosis activates the release of endorphins. If so, then naloxone should reverse the effects of hypnotically induced analgesia. However, the majority of studies that have looked at this have concluded that hypnotic analgesia is not dependent on endogenous opioid systems (Crawford and Gruzelier, 1992) An alternative explanation for the mechanism by which hypnosis acts is that of belief in efficacy (Wadden and Anderton, 1982). This suggests that hypnosis may be having a type of placebo effect but that this arises when it is perceived as a means to enable an existing procedure (such as therapy, surgery or drugs) to work. In these cases hypnosis may act to enhance the effectiveness of other treatment rather than to relieve pain or other symptoms itself.

This last possibility is consistent with the view that hypnosis is most effective when used alongside other techniques such as cognitive behavioural therapy (Kirsch *et al.*, 1995). Oakley *et al.* (1996) observe that, in itself, hypnosis is not a form of therapy. Rather, it can be used as an adjunct – providing a context in which therapies can be delivered more effectively. Hence they reject the use of labels such as 'hypnotherapy'; being an effective therapist must be the starting point from which the additional deployment of hypnosis may be advantageous to clients.

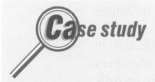

Case study

Anxiety and pain

Emma is a 42 year-old woman with a keen interest in running. She has participated in a number of sporting events and has been training to run in a marathon. However, over the last 6 months she has developed pain in her heels and her calves. Emma has been taking medication to relieve her pain and has also been treated by a podiatrist. However, her recovery isn't as fast as she had hoped and she has become extremely fearful and anxious that she will be unable to compete in the marathon. She tells her podiatrist that she has trouble sleeping, thinks about her condition a lot and is acutely aware of any signs of pain, and that her pain is worse when she is in a negative frame of mind. The podiatrist advises Emma that she should try some techniques to learn to relax and refers Emma back to her GP for further advice.

1 Which psychological factors are potentially contributing to the patient's pain?

2 How might pain theory help to explain the contribution of these psychological factors to pain?

3 What additional psychological treatment options might help the patient to cope with her pain?

KEY POINT

A patient may cope with pain with one or more of the following:

- anaesthesia, e.g. in surgery
- analgesia, e.g. using medication
- reduced awareness e.g. through hypnosis
- increased tolerance e.g. through distraction or relaxation.

CONCLUSIONS

Pain can be defined and, with variable reliability and validity, be measured in clinical settings and researched. The most commonly used tool for measuring pain is the McGill Pain Questionnaire, which assesses the intensity, location and emotional components of pain but does not differentiate well between different types of pain.

The gate control theory and especially its extension, the neuromatrix theory, offer an effective explanation of pain that accounts for the roles of pain specific neurons, the spinal cord and a range of physical, emotional, behavioural and cognitive factors that can increase or decrease perception of pain. The exact mechanism by which the gate and the moderating variables operate is still unclear, although evidence suggests a critical role for endorphins – natural opiate-like molecules. Endorphins appear also to be implicated in acupuncture and the placebo effect, although apparently not in hypnotic analgesia. Psychological variables of anxiety, conditioning, expectancy and cognitive dissonance all affect the perception of pain and they, too, relate to the placebo effect.

Patients' experience of pain depends on many factors, including their locus of control and deployment of emotion or problem-focused coping strategies. Physical interventions to reduce pain include analgesic medication, physical stimulation and surgery. Psychological strategies to enhance coping with pain including relaxation, biofeedback and hypnosis, have been shown to be effective for some patients and are becoming increasingly acceptable, in part because of the insight offered by these theories.

Reflective activity

Imagine that you wake up one morning with a headache. Make a list of actions you could take that, according to the gate control theory, would make it better or worse. If you choose either to sit and think positively 'Maybe it will go soon' or to get up and fetch some paracetamol, are you behaving in an emotion-focused or problem-focused way? Think about the way you actually respond to having a headache. Does your behaviour reflect an internal locus of control, suggesting that you believe that you can do something about the pain, or an external locus, believing that the progress of the headache is beyond your control?

RAPID RECAP

Check your progress so far by working through each of the following questions.

1 Describe one way in which pain is measured in a clinical setting and one way in which it can be measured for the purposes of research.

2 Too much work on a computer or reading a book can lead to an eye-strain headache. How would the gate control theory of pain account for the effectiveness of rubbing one's eyes to relieve the pain?

3 Vinar (1969) reported a case study of an individual who had become dependent upon a placebo. Use the idea of expectation to explain how this situation might have arisen.

If you have difficulty with any more of the questions, read through the section again to refresh your understanding before moving on.

KEY REFERENCES

Other references are listed on the supporting website.

Burns, E., Zobbi, V., Panzeri, D., Oskrochi, R. and Regalia, A. (2007) Aromatherapy in childbirth: a pilot randomised controlled trial. BJOG; 114: 838–844.

Engwall, M. and Sorensen Duppils, G. (2009) Music as a Nursing Intervention for Postoperative Pain: A Systematic Review. American Society of Peri-Anesthesia Nursing, 24(6): 370–83.

Levine, J.D., Gordon, N.C. and Fields, H.L. (1979) The role of endorphins in placebo analgesia. In: *Advances in Pain Research and Therapy*, vol. 3

(eds J.J. Bonica, J.C. Liebeskind and D. Albe-Fessard). New York Raven Press, New York.

Puntillo, K., Neighbor, M., O'Neil, N. and Nixon, R. (2003) Accuracy of emergency nurses in assessment of patients' pain. Pain Management Nursing, Dec;4(4): 171–5.

Shiri, S., Feintuch, U., Weiss, N., Pustilnik, A., Geffen, T., Kay, B., Meiner, Z. and Berger, I. (2013) A virtual reality system combined with biofeedback for treating pediatric chronic headache–a pilot study. Pain Medicine, 14(5): 621–7.

CHAPTER 9

BEREAVEMENT AND GRIEF

LEARNING OBJECTIVES

By the end of this chapter you should be able to:

- describe common experiences of bereaved individuals and the tasks of the grieving process

- understand differences in the grieving process between individuals, including social and cultural differences

- explain the experience of grieving from different theoretical perspectives

- identify ways in which bereaved individuals and health and social care staff can be supported when a patient dies.

I ndividuals differ in their experience and expression of grief and in the time they take to come to terms with the loss. In addition, differences in responses to bereavement may arise out of culturally determined patterns of behaviour following a death. Such differences must be respected, yet health and social care staff must be vigilant to detect individuals for whom grieving extends beyond the typical range of experience in terms of emotional extremes or time. This chapter considers first some generalizations that have been made about grieving including common individual and social differences and unusual, pathological, patterns of grief. Nurses are exposed to more death than virtually any other professional group so need to be prepared to offer help to the bereaved. Conversely, such constant contact with death can be stressful and health and social care professionals need support services too.

> **Grief**
> The emotional reaction to bereavement

> **Bereavement**
> The experience of the death of a person whom an individual knows closely

THE PROCESS OF BEREAVEMENT

The health and social care service aims to promote, sustain and recover the health of patients. Although sometimes inevitable, it is nevertheless distressing when this process cannot succeed and a patient dies. As a consequence, health and social care staff, who may themselves be affected by the death, are called upon to inform bereaved relatives and offer them support in their grief.

In addition to the suffering of grief, the bereaved may have other issues to cope with such as arranging a funeral and dealing with the dead person's personal effects. These are not of immediate consequence to health psychology, although, as a source of stress, the death of a loved one has health implications in itself so such responsibilities can add to the burden, negatively affecting the health of the bereaved. The impact of stress on bereavement is indicated by the greater debilitation of those who are bereaved through traumatic circumstances, such as after sudden or violent deaths (Kristensen et al., 2012).

Gerra et al. (2003) measured a range of variables in healthy participants who experienced an acute emotional stressor (such as the sudden death of a loved one) and non-stressed controls. They found that the individuals who had experienced the severe stressor reported more psychological distress and had impaired immune responses. As we saw earlier, such findings could account for the increased risk of illness experienced by the bereaved. Interestingly, Gerra et al. also found individual differences in both psychological and immune responses, with some bereaved participants experiencing more prolonged psychological and physiological symptoms. This, again, echoes the individual differences in coping described previously.

Bereaved people are themselves at greater risk of dying. Roelfs et al. (2013) conducted a meta-analysis of studies of the effects of the death of a spouse and found that people who had lost their spouse had a 22 per cent higher risk of dying relative to married people, even when factors, such as age were taken into account. This was more pronounced in men than in women. Furthermore, Rostila et al. (2013) found a similar effect in adults (aged 40–61) on the loss of a sibling, with the risk of mortality being elevated for about 6 years.

Although such findings may have indirect causes, such as loss of social support or the simple consequences of being alone, such as having a greater workload or being unable to afford healthy foods, the impact on health was clearly demonstrated in Rostila et al.'s study, which focused on subsequent risk of death through myocardial infarction. Kemminki and Li (2003) explored cancer risks following loss of a spouse. Cancers of various parts of the digestive system were increased in widows and widowers, and lung cancer was higher in widowers. These findings were explained by differences in exposure to carcinogens and poor nutrition. The increased lung cancer in widowers reflects their higher tobacco smoking and increased upper aerodigestive cancer in both genders can be explained by increased alcohol and tobacco use. Greater oesophageal cancer in men may be accounted for by diet, as women may have more cooking experience and eat more vegetables than men. People are likely to drink more following bereavement and this may account for the increased prevalence of cirrhosis of the liver in widows, and widowers (Mellström et al., 1982; Stroebe and Stroebe, 1983).

Aerodigestive tract
The organs and tissues of the respiratory system and upper parts of the digestive system (lips, mouth, tongue, nose, throat, vocal cords, oesophagus and windpipe)

Symptoms of grief

Physical symptoms	Cognitive symptoms
Tightness in the throat	Denial
Breathlessness and the need to sigh	Difficulty concentrating
Feeling of hollowness or emptiness	Memory problems
Feeling of hollowness or emptiness	Dreams of the deceased
Bodily aches and pains	Hallucinations of the deceased
	Preoccupation with the deceased

Behavioural symptoms	Emotional symptoms
Appetite changes	Numbness
Sleep disturbance	Sadness
Repetitious behaviour	Anger
Social withdrawal	Guilt
Carrying reminders of the deceased	Depression
Avoiding reminders of the dead	Yearning
Searching for the deceased	Loneliness
Crying	Helplessness
Restlessness	Relief
Reminiscing	
Laughing	

Grief is a normal, universal reaction, which serves as an adaptation to the new situation in which an individual finds themselves after the loss of someone close to them. Grief reactions vary, and some variations fall outside the anticipated range in terms of duration or severity. Acute grief is the initial, painful response and integrated grief is the ongoing adaptation to the death but in some cases complicated (or pathological) grief arises, in which the 'acute grief' response is unusually intense, prolonged or unresolved (Tal Young *et al.*, 2012).

Delayed grief may arise when the loss is ignored or denied but eventually accepted. This can occur if grieving is difficult, such as for a parent who loses a partner but suppresses his or her feelings to ease the loss experienced by their children. Sometimes grief may be absent when it would be expected. A Freudian interpretation of absent grief would suggest that the absence of grief would arise from repression, which, could lead to later psychological symptoms such as neurosis. Although there is evidence to support the idea of repression in general (e.g. Koehler *et al.*, 2002), the relationship with pathological grief is only assumed and there is a growing body of evidence to suggest that resilience, i.e. the absence of pathological grief, even after traumatic losses, is surprisingly common (Mancini and Bonnano, 2006). Indeed, Bonnano (2004) observed that research is often based on those who seek help, so resilient individuals are underrepresented and, furthermore, that except those experiencing the most traumatic losses, grief therapy may actually be detrimental.

Only about 10 per cent of bereaved individuals experience chronic grief (Bonnano and Kaltman, 2001) although this is more common after violent

Repression
A state in which access to traumatic memories is prevented. Freud suggests that they remain in the unconscious – in order to protect the individual's conscious awareness – but such memories can consequentially cause disturbances to mental health

Neurosis
A state of unrealistic anxiety

deaths (Kaltman and Bonnano, 2003) and when a child dies (Bonnano *et al.*, 2005). From a review of such evidence, Bonanno and Mancini (2008) concluded that given the prevalence of resilience to bereavement, psychotherapeutic interventions should be reserved for those in most need. However, this does not detract from the need for support to ensure that those who are resilient cope well, hence the need for nurses to be aware of the grief process and the needs of grieving family, friends and colleagues.

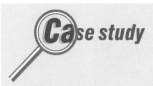

Holding it all together

Mr Davidson (John) is 42 years-old and the father of two teenage sons, Christopher 18 years-old and Patrick 14 years-old. His wife and mother of the children died 6 months ago from cervical cancer. The prognosis was poor and advanced at the time of diagnosis and she was dead in less than a year. John has found it very difficult to come to terms with his new situation. He has returned to work but does little else. Christopher is about to begin University. He had promised his Mum he would continue with his dream of becoming a lawyer. Patrick however, has been causing problems at school. John is at his wits end and is dreading Christopher moving away

to live in a flat near his university although he knows this is necessary and he is proud of him. He has no idea what to do about Patrick. He makes an appointment for his GP, third in 6 weeks as he has been having problems with headaches and indigestion. John is reluctant to take time off work as his employers had been very supportive following the death of his wife, although his GP had recommended that he needed to be off. On this occasion, and while telling the GP his symptoms, John suddenly becomes emotional.

1 Why do you think the GP has recommended John take time off work?

2 Do you think there could be other reasons why John is reluctant to take time off work?

3 What could the GP do to make the patient feel he could confide in her?

Returning to complicated grief, this is characterized by its duration and distress. Intense longing interferes with normal functioning and making it difficult for the individual to re-establish a meaningful life in the absence of the deceased. They may be plagued by recurrent images of their loved one, be unable to retrieve any positive memories or the strength of their yearning may lead them to thoughts of suicide. Individuals themselves bereaved through suicide are amongst those who experience complicated grief (Young *et al.*, 2012), as are those who lose loved ones through sudden or violent deaths, such as in cases of murder, military losses or victims of disaster (Kristensen *et al.*, 2012).

Health Care Professional

General Practitioner

A more frequent visitor

Mr John Davidson rarely visited the surgery prior to his wife becoming terminally ill. Even then he never came to the surgery about himself, instead only if his wife required to be seen or to collect a prescription for her. Recently he has been a frequent visitor with varying physical symptoms which on consideration, and although real for him, I suspect are a consequence of his bereavement. It is not unusual for grief to present in a physical manner and I am hoping that as we have a good relationship, I can persuade him to start talking to me about how he is really feeling. I also know a little of the problems he is having with his younger son, which is causing him a great deal of stress. This type of behaviour, including anger, in his son, may also be a consequence of the loss of his mother and ideally I would like to suggest that they all meet with a family therapist at the local hospice.

Describing the bereavement process

Grief follows bereavement but its exact pattern depends on the bereaved individual, the nature of the death and the characteristic mourning of the society. Some individuals experience little grief – for example, those people who feel that the death represents a relief from suffering for the dead person (although this is not always the case in such circumstances). For most bereaved people, the grieving process may last for weeks, months or even years. During the early stages, the bereaved can expect considerable social support, offering both emotional solace and practical help. However, when this ceases the grieving process is rarely over and the bereaved person may feel very lonely with neither their loved one nor the previous level of social support. This sense of abandonment and isolation is exemplified in the following passage: 'Grief following bereavement by death is aggravated if the person lost is the person to whom one would turn in times of trouble. Faced with the biggest trouble she has ever had, the widow repeatedly finds herself turning toward the person who is not there' (Parkes, 2000, p. 327).

Early approaches to the scientific study of grief included generalized descriptions of the process through a series of stages, such as those of Kübler-Ross (1969) and Parkes (1972). However, people vary in their experience of grief in many ways: whether they experience the symptoms in the order suggested, or at all, as well as in the exact nature of their experience and how long it lasts. An alternative approach was to identify the tasks to be achieved through mourning. Worden (1991) proposed that these were:

- accepting the reality of the loss
- working through the pain

Mourning
The socially and culturally dictated ways of expressing grief is influenced by culturally determined rituals.

- adjusting to the absence of the deceased from the environment
- moving forward in life.

Even within this wider remit individual differences arise, with people taking differing lengths of time over some tasks or failing to achieve them at all. Indeed, this is one way in which complicated grief can be identified.

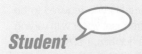

Student

Student Health Visitor

Dealing with grief

I felt really nervous when the health visitor said one of the GP's was willing to let me sit in and observe her surgery that morning although she would have to get consent from each patient as they arrived in her room. Although it was all very interesting, the case that stuck in my mind was the patient who started to tell the doctor about the problems he was having with his stomach but then he just stopped speaking and looked like he might cry. I felt really uncomfortable as this was a man in his forties and the doctor had not had the time to give me his background prior to him being seen. Although the patient was in the surgery for just 15 minutes, I learned so much. The doctor just sat silent facing the patient and saying nothing. She gently put her hand on his arm and waited a while before saying that she was glad he was allowing his feelings to surface. There wasn't much said at all but she arranged for him to come back the next day for a longer time when she hoped he would start talking to her about the loss of his wife who died a year before.

Two models of grieving

Kübler–Ross (1969) proposed a five stage process of adjusting to death:

- denial
- anger
- bargaining
- depression
- acceptance.

Parkes (1972) identified four phases of mourning:

- numbness
- yearning and denial
- disorganization and despair
- reorganization.

According to such models, a bereaved person is likely to initially experience pain, numbness or desolation. Through this 'haze' they may deny that the loss is real or permanent. Such feelings are common and often intense; they may feel unable to think or do anything and cannot contemplate ever feeling differently. Health and social care professionals need to be aware that this detachment from reality is common and does not represent a genuine failure to accept that their loved one is dead.

Simultaneously, or subsequently, the bereaved individual may experience strong feelings of guilt and/or anger. They may blame themselves for the death, or resent the dead person for leaving them. They may 'bargain', trying to find ways to reverse the loss. Again, this stage has the potential to present health and social care staff with problems as they may feel drawn into the bereaved person's essentially private crisis.

During this early period of grief, an important marker may be a leave-taking ceremony, such as a funeral. This allows the bereaved to make a statement of farewell to the deceased. The ritual, by dictating behaviour through formalities, may be helpful because it both contains emotion and allows for the expression of those feelings. There are gender differences here, with women benefiting as the funeral may represent a transition to a more senior family role or boost confidence through successfully organizing the event. For men, however, a funeral may be a hurdle, if they feel displaying emotion is inappropriate but doubt that they can fulfil this social convention.

Whilst depression and despair may arise during grief, these reactions are not inevitable, although crying and intense sadness are very common. Conversely, it is not the case that there is an absolute absence of positive emotions. Lund *et al.* (2008) (see Research in Brief) found that bereaved spouses experienced positive emotions, and perceived this to be important. Women more than men may find that they need to continuously replay events surrounding the death – a process called obsessional review. The loved one is recalled in a positive light, which may provide a way to come to terms with the death.

RESEARCH IN BRIEF

Lund, DA *et al.* (2008) Humor, Laughter & Happiness in the Daily Lives of Recently Bereaved Spouses.

Aim: To investigate the importance of positive emotions for the bereft.

Procedure: The participants were 292 men (39 per cent) and women (61 per cent) age 50 who had been recently widowed (5–24 weeks). They were asked about both how important they perceived positive emotions (humour, laughter and happiness) to be and about their actual experience of positive emotions in their daily lives.

Results: Most participants rated humour and happiness as important in their daily lives and that they were experiencing these emotions more than expected. Experiencing positive emotions was associated with better adjustment to bereavement (lower grief and depression). This was the case regardless of the extent to which the bereaved person valued having those emotions although race and the unexpectedness of the death were important.

Conclusion: Positive emotions are important, even soon after the loss. There are cultural differences in expectation and acceptability of positive emotions during bereavement although in general, they are beneficial for most people and can be seen in the context of the Dual Process Model (DPM) as oriented towards restoration.

Ultimately, the bereaved individual should start to cope as they restructure their life in the absence of their loved one. Even in cases where the death has been anticipated this may take many months, in part because cultural norms dictate that it is 'improper' to prepare for a death and in part because such situations may be fraught with regret or self-blame. In relationships where each person played a distinct role, the bereaved individual learns a new set of skills such as household or financial management. The establishment of a new relationship may be difficult to consider for the bereaved person or for others to accept.

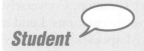

Student

Final year nursing student

A first experience of a patient dying …

'I remember the nurse I was working with when I had to care for a patient who had died for the first time in my career. She suggested that I talk to the deceased person as I might normally, but I felt a bit uncomfortable about this. I do feel that this is a really important job, doing the last thing for them in as peaceful way as possible. I find it is much harder if I have known the patient for a long time, as it is more upsetting when you have to lay this person out.'

Reflective activity

If you have experienced the death of a patient on a placement, can you identify any of these stages in the relatives, other patients on the ward or staff?

The Dual Process Model

So far we have looked at descriptive, stage-like, models of grieving which help us to understand generalizations that can be made about common experiences in the grief process. Many of original assumptions on which these were based have been challenged:

- Stages/tasks may not all be experienced, may arise in different orders or may be repeated.
- The norm is considered to be resilience rather than depression – which is much less common than previously assumed (Wortman and Silver, 1989).
- Freud's notion that grieving should result in detachment has been replaced by an acceptance of the role of a continuing bond with the deceased (Klass *et al.*, 1996).
- The need to 'work through' grief, or for formal support, is no longer believed to be desirable for all (Bonanno and Mancini, 2008).

More recently, research has focused on the extent to which an explanation of grieving can allow for an interchange between states rather than a linear progression from a negative position to a positive one. The **Dual Process Model** of Coping with Bereavement, see Table 9.1, (Stroebe and Schut, 1999) aimed not only to integrate these two aspects but do develop a way to predict the likelihood of a successful outcome from grieving. This model proposes that grief is a dynamic process rather than a linear one. Instead of progressing through orderly stages and emerging with a resolution, the bereft fluctuate between two different coping strategies.

The loss orientation refers to the individual's focus on processing their feelings and thoughts about their loss and the behaviours that arise from these. This is illustrated, for example, by the painful dwelling on or searching for the lost loved one. In contrast, the restoration orientation refers to their emotions, cognitions and behaviours surrounding the recognition of and attempts to deal with the changes that need to be made. Thus at any time an individual might be overwhelmed by feelings of abandonment, memories of the way things were, or crying. Such aspects are loss-oriented and relate to the mental appraisal of the loss and the eventual acceptance of it. Restoration orientation is reflected in emotional satisfaction of resolving a practical issue relating to the death, cognitive strategies including distraction from the sense of suffering and new behaviours might include accepting new roles or new ways to cope.

According to Stroebe and Schut, this oscillation offers a way to cope with the loss by moderating the suffering of grief by alternately exploring the loss and the future. Importantly, this allows for the distinction between the process of coping and the consequences of that process, i.e. whether the outcomes are adaptive or maladaptive. Note that although there is a superficial similarity between these two orientations and the emotion versus

Loss orientation
One of psychological perspectives an individual may have during grieving, which focuses on the absence of their loved one and its negative consequences

Restoration orientation
One of psychological perspectives an individual may have during grieving, which focuses on the changes needed to progress with one's life after the loss of a loved one

problem-focused coping strategies, they are different. For example, some aspects of the loss orientation can inevitably only be dealt with by emotionally-focused strategies (such as an acceptance that the deceased cannot be brought back, since this is unchangeable). However, others may be more effectively tackled with problem-focused coping, such as the need to continue to feel close to the deceased being aided by planting a tree in their memory, which can be visited and tended. Similarly, an emotion-focused strategy (e.g. of ignoring the bills) or a problem-focused one (of seeing the bank manager) may be used to cope with aspects of restoration, such as dealing with the financial situation.

In practice, the DPM can explain why a grieving person may sometimes seem accepting of the loss and on other occasions seem to be denying or avoiding it. For nurses, this provides the reassurance that whilst having to see a bereaved individual suffering is painful, this expression is a focus on the loss orientation and is necessary for grief work but will alternate with the opposing position, the resolution orientation, during which they will attempt to overcome the secondary losses associated with the death and that both of these are crucial parts of the process of adjustment. To focus purely on the loss prevents the individual dealing with the secondary losses. Conversely, whilst a focus on restoration helps to sustain coping, and is necessary for moving on, to never confront the loss would prevent the individual from coming to terms with their grief. Bennett *et al.* (2010) found that individuals who were coping well with grief exhibited a balance between loss-orientation, such as experiencing grief as a continuing bond, and restoration-orientation, such as coping with new roles, identities and relationships. Those individuals adjusting less well reported more stressors, such as the denial or avoidance of restoration changes, and more loss-oriented distraction or avoidance of grief.

Table 9.1 According to the Dual Process Model, the bereft oscillate between the two orientations

Loss orientation	Restoration orientation
Grief work	Dealing with life changes, such as coping with things you hadn't done before, such as washing, house maintenance, finances, etc.
Intrusion of grief, e.g. crying	Finding distractions from grief
Letting go or relocating ties	Doing new things
Denial of restoration changes	Denial/avoidance of grief
Avoidance of restoration changes	Establishing new roles, relationships and identities

Compared to earlier models of grieving, this model is better able to account for individual differences in grieving. Since it does not indicate a specific pathway for grief, or stress one process over another, it can explain a wide range of grieving patterns, as considered in the next section.

Continuing bonds theory

The processes and models that we have considered so far aim, in different ways, to explain bereavement in terms of the cessation of a relationship. Indeed, all have largely stressed the need for grief to lead to emotional disengagement. In contrast, continuing bonds theory suggests that the bereaved person maintains an attachment to their loved one, i.e. that despite the physical separation an emotional tie continues. Hogan and DeSantis (1992) studied bereavement in adolescents who had lost a sibling. They found that, when asked the question 'If you could ask or tell your dead sibling something, what would it be?' They typically replied 'I miss you and I love you'. Their answers were in the present tense, regardless of how long ago the sibling had died. This suggests that they had an ongoing attachment long after the sibling's death. Subsequent studies have demonstrated similarly enduring links to lost parents and siblings in children and partners and children in adults. For example, Silverman et al. (1992) showed that bereaved children and adolescents retained a connection to their deceased parent. They developed an internal construction of the dead parent and this altered relationship was preserved as they grew up. Field and Friedrichs (2004) investigated the continuing bond of women following the death of a husband. With longer times since bereavement, the widows showed a stronger relationship between coping based on a continuing bond, and positive mood.

Klass et al. (1996) proposed the theory of continuing bonds based on studies of bereaved parents. The findings showed that parents maintained bonds with their dead children, for example with the children being important in conversation. The adults reconstructed their relationships in a way that was meaningful to them, e.g. through links to objects, such as the child's possessions and through rituals that evoked memories of the child. The theory suggests that to preserve a sense of the relationship with the dead person is natural and healthy. It is achieved by developing an inner representation of the dead person which replaces the living reality and so provides a vehicle for the bereaved person's love of and need for the person they have lost without denying that loss. The challenge for those who support the bereaved is therefore to find ways to help them to hold and adapt the continuing relationship in new and different ways, rather than trying to separate themselves from it.

Packman et al. (2006) suggest key clinical implications for young people bereaved of siblings. Encouraging the continuing bond is important, as is the recognition that whilst in some respects the parent is the best placed to do this, but in practice that they too are bereft. Other people, such as relatives, friends and health and social carers may be important in offering a window for expression, allowing open talk about the deceased, especially at significant events such as birthdays or starting a new school. Enabling practical strategies such as carrying a photograph or wearing the dead sibling's clothes may be helpful as it can facilitate fond memories rather than focusing on sad ones. Importantly, whilst suggestions and opportunities can be given, the connection cannot be made *for* the child. Each grieving individual must build their own attachment within the new reality. Finally, for some children, such as those who endured an abusive or manipulative relationship with their deceased sibling, it may be unwise to advocate the maintenance of the bond.

Individual differences in grieving

It is worth observing that there will be differences in the way that even a single death is experienced because those close to the deceased will have had different relationships with them. The loss of one's parents represents a loss of the past. Losing a partner is the loss of the present. For the parent who loses a child, their future is lost. Beyond this difference in perspective, differences arise due to many factors including gender, age, personality and the circumstances of the death. When the individual cannot talk to others about the death, or there are feelings of guilt or shame, bereavement is much harder, for example, following still births (Cacciatore, 2013), when a child with disabilities dies (Todd, 2007) and for people with disabilities who are, themselves, bereaved (Read and Elliot, 2007). Some of these issues are explored in the following sections.

Gender differences

Women tend to display more overt grief than men. However, they are also more likely to benefit from attending a funeral and are less likely to turn to alcohol than men. There are also gender differences in the *way* that bereavement is experienced. Following the death of a partner, women describe feelings of abandonment whereas men describe feeling dismembered. For heterosexual couples this can be understood in terms of the meaning of marriage for women – as a key social relationship. So, for a widow, returning to work may help to satisfy the loss of her interpersonal relationship. Emotional responses also differ between widows and widowers: women tend to feel angry and cry, wanting someone to sort their life out for them, whereas men feel 'choked up' and guilty. Although they are better at accepting the death of their partner in some respects, making a faster social recovery, widowers take longer to overcome the emotional consequences. The DPM explains this difference as a focus on loss-orientation by women but on restoration-orientation by men. As a generalization, this difference works well for heterosexual couples, unless one or other is so extreme that there is no oscillation (Stroebe and Schut, 2010). For nurses, it may be helpful to recognize this difference, for example, in parents who have lost a child. Whilst the mother may feel of the father that 'he is grieving less than me', this can alternatively be understood as 'he is grieving differently from me'.

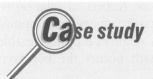

Unrecognized grief

Individuals may have reasons for choosing not to disclose a loving, close, same sex relationship. Not being 'out' can have huge implications for couples in same sex relationships when one partner dies.

Jeremy and his partner David had not disclosed their relationship to anyone. Jeremy said David had been very clear they could not be open about their relationship. When David died his family made the funeral arrangements in which Jeremy had no say:

> 'I knew he wanted to be buried next to his mother. He ended up being cremated the other side of the city and cremation was totally against his religion...I couldn't stop them but it was like strangers organizing his funeral; I was his family...But he never wanted it to be known that he was gay. And I respected that, so he wasn't out, I wasn't out either. I couldn't talk to my family...they thought David was just a friend. I was a right mess. I had no-one to turn to.'

Another gay man, Michael, recalls a friend who did not get compassionate leave when his partner died and very little recognition of his loss other than from close friends:

> 'I went to his funeral and the family were none too happy with the situation, I don't think they wanted people knowing their son, brother, was gay. And my friend who was grieving, he's been with his partner for years, he never got a mention from the vicar, not one.'

The significance of Jeremy's loss and grief is not only not recognized and validated but is further complicated by the absence of personal networks where he may have found support and by David's family taking over. In the second case, Michael describes how his friend, the bereaved partner, received some recognition from friends but none from his partner's family, who refused to acknowledge the relationship.

In the past health and social care staff may have demonstrated overt, if not deliberate, homophobic behaviour. Evidence does now present a more optimistic picture, for example, Erlen *et al.* (1999) found a very low incidence of homophobic attitudes among nurses (an average score of 1.14 on a range of 0–28). However, even recent evidence suggests that lesbian, gay, bisexual and transgender (LGBT) people experience discrimination in the health service. For example, Almack *et al.* (2010) cites case studies of problematic end-of-life care and difficult grief, and even civil partners sometimes encounter difficulties in achieving recognition (RCN/UNISON: 'Not "Just" a Friend'). Although a homosexual relationship may have been long and committed, the remaining individual may not be, or may not want to be, acknowledged by their partner's family. Thus, the grieving survivor will be just as emotionally distressed as a heterosexual partner would be but may be excluded from activities that form an important part of the grieving process (such as the funeral or post-mortem, if there is one). Health and social care professionals need to be aware of this risk. Moss and Almack (2012) observe that the key issue is openness. Whilst nursing staff may wish to 'treat everyone the same', in practice this may not be appropriate and being open and letting an individual lead their own disclosures and express their needs is important, especially as many LGBT people may have had negative experiences elsewhere in their lives.

Gay couples may, however, be advantaged in one respect in relation to heterosexuals. McDougall (1993) reviewed the literature on ageing in homosexual men and women and found that, because gay relationships are flexible in the roles that each individual takes, when death occurs the bereaved individual may cope better.

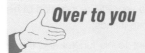

Over to you

Can an LGBT person's partner, whether they are in a civil partnership or not, be nominated as their 'next-of-kin' or 'point of contact'?

Adjusting to traumatic deaths

Grieving is less pronounced following the death of an elderly compared to a younger person. This difference may arise because of the unexpected nature of death in the young. Similarly, in traumatic deaths, such as accidents or suicide, grief is more intense. In such situations, both men and women experience more difficulties in coming to terms with their loss. The grief of parents who lose a child is typically intense and may adversely affect their mental health (Rogers *et al.*, 2008). This is particularly so when the death is violent (Dyregrov *et al., 2003). Nakajima* et al. (2012) reviewed studies of complicated grief and reported that whilst in the general population it is experienced by about 2–7 per cent of those who lose significant others, this rises to as much as 78 per cent following violent deaths. For example, 21.9 per cent after homicide and traffic accidents and 43.2 per cent following the September 11th attacks.

RESEARCH IN BRIEF

Dyregrov *et al.* (2003) Predictors of psychosocial stress after suicide

Aim: To investigate differences in distress experienced by parents whose young children die through suicide, sudden infant death syndrome (SIDS) or accident.

Procedure: The distress experienced by 232 parents from 140 families bereaved by traumatic death (suicide, SIDS or accident) was investigated one-and-a-half years after the loss.

Findings: More than half of the participants were still suffering grief reactions. There were no significant differences between parents of children who had lost a child through suicide or through accident, although both showed greater distress than parents bereaved by SIDS. The best predictor of distress was social isolation.

Conclusion: Sudden and traumatic deaths of children have lasting effects on grieving parents, especially if they receive less social support.

Anticipatory grieving and the effects of caring

Pearlin *et al.* (1989) describe the feelings of anticipatory grieving experienced by people who care for Alzheimer's sufferers. They identify feelings of loss resembling bereavement while the individual is still alive because the person they once knew no longer exists. Such caregivers may experience emotions including anger, fear of abandonment as the relationship deteriorates, depression and sleeplessness. Physiological changes in anticipatory grief, including immunosuppression, have also be identified. If carers themselves have good social support, they tend to cope better but, in general, the subsequent grief of those who are caregivers for a long time is likely to be problematic (Shultz *et al.*, 2008). Clukey (2003) interviewed carers experiencing anticipatory grieving in relation to a family member. She described additional emotions, including sadness, feeling overwhelmed or trapped, frustration and guilt. These closely reflect the experiences of grief after a death. Richardson (2010) used the DPM to explore grieving in older adults and found that, in general, restoration orientation was helpful, allowing the individual to benefit from social interactions. However, she also found that the effects of caregiving prior to the death of a spouse has an adverse affect on well-being, which may be in part due to the reduction in social contacts (who could be helpful after the death) during the time-consuming process of caring. Contrary to expectations from the DPM, for these individuals, joining a club post-bereavement made them less rather than more happy suggesting that different restoration activities satisfy different needs.

> **Anticipatory grieving**
> Emotions experienced because of a predicted loss, such as when a patient has a terminal illness. Although it can help an individual to prepare for the impending death, the prolonged process of separation can worsen emotional coping

Cultural differences in grieving

Many societies have clear cultural rituals for responding to bereavement. Whilst some of these may be more positive than others – celebrating the dead person's life rather than mourning their death – a socially determined pattern of responses can help to make grieving easier. The presence of social guidelines for the bereaved and those with whom they come into contact reduces stress. Walter *et al.* (2000) suggest that, in Britain, traditionally explicit expectations about the behaviour of grieving people do not exist; no longer are widows expected to dress in black and wear a veil nor widowers to wear a black armband.

In some cultures, however, such conventions guide the expression of grief in the bereaved. The Irish wake, which may include a feast, allows the body to be watched by relatives for several days until the burial. In contrast, the customs surrounding bereavement for orthodox Jews determine when the bereaved leave the house, how they dress and when recreation can be enjoyed. Exactly 1 year after the death, mourning is completed by the dedication of the tombstone. Traditional Japanese death rituals aim to enable the deceased to travel to a better place. Loved ones assist this journey with ceremonies, ritual bathing of the corpse and a feast that returns the mourners to the community. The Hindu religion views life and death as a cycle; thus death is a transitional state before rebirth.

The absence of tradition and the 'stiff upper lip' attitude prevalent in Britain (and in America), in which the role of the bereaved in dealing with the practicalities of the death is much reduced, may not, ultimately, benefit everyone trying to come to terms with a loss. So, when health and social care professionals encounter bereaved individuals they must consider their cultural as well as individual needs in terms of expressing their grief. The DPM can be useful in this context. Wikan (1988) provides contrasting examples of the Muslim communities. On the island of Bali where behaviour is highly restoration-oriented, there are few outward expressions of grief and following a death, daily life continues as normal. whereas Muslims in Egypt express their grief openly, publically reminiscing and sharing their anguish – the loss-orientation.

Children's experience of bereavement

As adults we expect, ultimately, that we will experience bereavement but bereavement during childhood is also surprisingly common. One in 30 children will have experienced the death of a parent by the time they are 19 and their response to this experience is different from that of adults. Children suffer many of the same emotions, of guilt, anger, numbness and depression, but their response is less predictable than that of adults.

Another important difference between children and adults is the child's differing understanding of the concept of death. Nagy (1948) described three developmental stages in a child's comprehension of the meaning of death:

- **Age 3 to 5 years** – death as separation or a diminished form of life, a reversible state like sleeping.
- **Age 5–6 to 9 years** – death as final, a permanent state but one that can be avoided and is neither universal nor personal.
- **Age 10** – death as universal and inevitable, including the child's own eventual death.

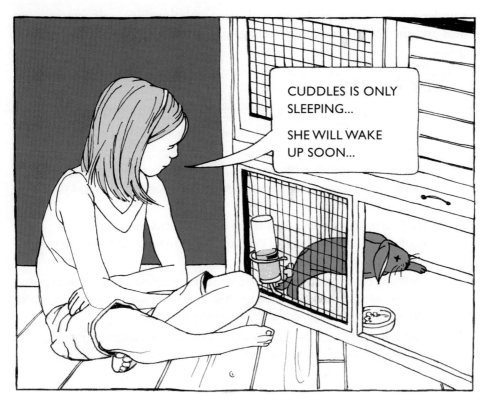

Age affects understanding of death.

Although the exact ages will vary with individual children, the general pattern of progressive understanding has been supported by subsequent research. It is important for health and social carers who are working with bereaved children to recognize that they will have a concept of death and may need, as much as adults, to express and discuss their thoughts and feelings (Brookes, 2002).

Davis (1989) observed that children are often misinformed or uninformed about death and, as a consequence, are denied the right to grieve. Through art therapy, Davis suggests, children can be given permission to express their emotions without fear of disapproval. Using puppets, drawing, story telling and clay modelling, art therapy allows children to become aware of and display their feelings, work them through and enjoy the experience. Similarly, Roberts and McFerran (2013) demonstrated that through music therapy, bereaved children could address issues of their relationships and their loss.

The importance of enabling grieving in children does not end with reducing their immediate suffering. Ellis *et al.* (2013) have shown that the long-term effects of early parental death have much greater impact in adulthood if the child's grief is not well managed. They found that when appropriate social support for both the child and surviving parent is lacking and there is a failure to give clear and honest information that is relevant to the child's level of understanding later problems with trust, relationships, self-esteem, loneliness and the ability to express feelings can arise.

KEY POINTS

- Grief is a reaction to bereavement, it may be formalized through ritualistic mourning. Some people are more resilient than others, some suffer prolonged or complicated grief.

- Grief can be described in different ways, as stages (e.g. numbness, anger, bargaining, depression, acceptance) or tasks (e.g. accepting, working through, adjusting to the loss and moving on).

- The DPM suggests individuals alternate between a loss-orientation (e.g. focussing on the missing of the loved one) and a restoration orientation (dealing with the new situation).

- Continuing bonds theory suggests emotional disengagement from the dead person is neither necessary nor preferable and that a lasting attachment to them is normal and healthy, e.g. through conversation, objects or rituals.

- There are individual differences in the experience and expression of grief, e.g. differences in relation to gender, culture, age and the nature of the death (e.g. traumatic or anticipated).

HELPING BEREAVED INDIVIDUALS
Support for families

Imparting bad news is difficult; because it is hard to receive news of death, it is therefore hard to give. It is advisable to avoid sidestepping the issue, beginning with as little introductory information possible, perhaps just identifying health and social care staff present and their roles, then providing information about the death as gently as possible without disguising it – the message must be honest and open. Communication needs to be clear and consistent, the use of expressions such as 'expired' or 'no longer with us' are not helpful, they simply have the potential to lead to confusion.

Once individuals have learned of their loss they need support. Health and social care staff have a key role here. It is advisable to:

- listen to what is said
- stay calm
- accept the emotions that are displayed (such as anger or an absence of response in a silent recipient)
- give the bereaved person time to process the information given to them
- accept and not disguise your own sadness, without burdening them further.

It is also inadvisable to:

- attempt to explain how you feel or your previous experiences
- attempt to justify why this has happened.

Once the bereaved person has said all they want to, further assistance is important. Following a death, bereaved individuals are likely to be shocked and may find new tasks difficult. Health and social care staff can provide initial information and reassurance that many bereaved individuals will need about what will happen next. Such information will include:

- the need for a relative to take a copy of the death certificate issued by the doctor certifying the death to the Registrar of Births, Marriages and Deaths
- possibly the need for a post-mortem examination and, if so, the potential for delay in issuing a death certificate
- how to find an undertaker (without making specific recommendations).

Reassurance at this stage may include the need to:

- talk through a request for a post-mortem
- allay fears about mutilation of the dead person's body
- accept that undertakers can help the family with many organizational aspects of dealing with the death, not just organizing the funeral.

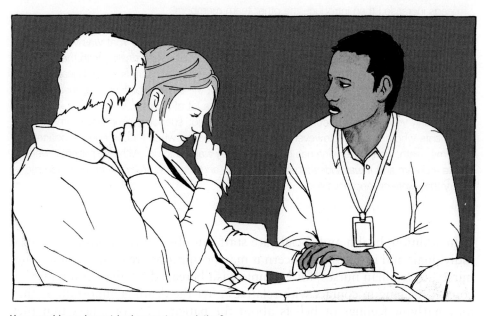

How would you impart bad news to a relative?

Responding to the bereft

Bruce (2007) summarizes three key attitudes for caregivers to remember.

Empathy: The simultaneous awareness of oneself and the other person

Attentiveness: Remaining 'tuned-in' – cognitively, emotionally and spiritually present for the individual, which requires significant personal reserves in difficult circumstances.

Respect: Openness and cultural sensitivity.

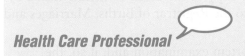

Health Care Professional

Community District Nurse

Caring for dying patients

'We can be involved with a family for weeks/months/years before somebody dies and during that time we've built up a relationship not just with the patient but with the husband, or wife, the children and the neighbours. We all put terminal patients at the top of the list. It's all part of case-load management and you get better at that by doing it.

I do all the initial assessments, and anything the other staff are unsure of. I get involved with the more complex cases, and the early stages of palliative care. People want to have one person going in that they have to relate to. It's not helpful to have various nurses popping in because they have to go over and over the same things. I do a lot of the early palliative care as it requires quite expert practice and as the physical care needs increase I then introduce the other team members.

It can be very tough, we had a really bad patch, we'd been busy all year with palliative care, and we had about four patients all very ill at the same time. That was very tough because we were trying to keep the patients symptom-free, and dealing with the grief is very time-consuming. That's when being part of an extended team is a help because we do try and help each other out. We all know about the terminal patients because we all cover them at the weekends. We give each other a lot of support.

I think you need to ensure a mix of patients. Not spending your whole time with patients who are dying. However, there is a satisfaction when it goes right. A peaceful home death, where everyone has done what they wanted to do. With one patient it went like a dream and it was indescribably satisfying, and the letter from the family made me cry they were so appreciative.'

In addition, health and social care staff can observe reactions of bereaved individuals and in cases of concern it may be appropriate to alert community nurses. Macmillan nurses, for example, visit bereaved relatives as a matter of course. Keeping in contact with relatives after the death is important as they may harbour feelings or beliefs about the patient's life or illness that they cannot come to terms with. Nurses may find that they are asked to help, for example taking away equipment or medicines that act as reminders of the loss. This can provide an opportunity to allow bereaved individuals to talk about their emotions or about their loved one.

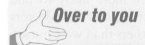

Over to you

Find out about the provision for bereaved people in your local area. Is bereavement counselling offered at your local hospitals or Macmillan hospice if you have one? Look at the advertisements in Yellow Pages for Funeral Services offered in your area. What range of services is provided? Do you have a local branch of Cruse? Does your own doctors' surgery have information about funeral directors? Finally, consider how aware someone might be of any of these services in the event of an unexpected death – how much of what you discovered was new to you?

Health and social care staff will have priorities of their own, such as removing personal belongings from the hospital, and these needs should be expressed with due consideration for the feelings of the bereaved individuals.

In the longer term, a range of services is available to people who have suffered bereavement and for those enduring anticipatory grieving. These include:

- individual counselling
- group therapy
- family therapy with the dying person in a hospice setting
- support groups of similarly affected individuals.

Some evidence suggests that such support is beneficial as it reduces the risk of subsequent psychological disorders. One way in which such services may be of use is in allowing the bereaved individual to 'work through' their grief. However, not all people desire such assistance and recent research on resilience suggests that formal support is not always necessary.

Other aspects of adjustment are the need to replace lost social support and to regain control. Many bereaved people throw themselves into work or new relationships following the loss of a loved one. By so doing, they may achieve replacement control or social support. Bereavement counselling should enable individuals to seek a workable balance between these needs. In the short term, counselling itself provides social support and encourages the individual to take control of their own existence, a strategy that will, in turn, lead to sources of social support.

Support for staff

Apart from servicemen and service women in wartime, nursing staff encounter death more often than people in any other profession. Wagner *et al.* (1997)

found that 76 per cent of nurses reported crying when at work and that the main cause was identification with the suffering of dying patients and their families. Vejlgaard and Addington-Hall (2005) studied perceptions of palliative/terminal care nurses. They found that nurses were more likely to find reward in working with dying patients than were doctors, and that doctors were more likely to leave the care of dying patients to others than were nurses. Unsurprisingly, the extent to which nurses are exposed to death can be stressful and traumatic.

Valente (2003) found that health and social care professionals were significantly affected by a patient's death by suicide, experiencing feelings of guilt and responsibility. Whilst Anderson and Gaugler (2006) found certified nursing assistants in nursing home settings, whose patients will inevitably die, suffered complicated grief, they also found that their experiences could lead to personal growth. Indeed, Moyle Wright and Hogan (2008) suggest that hospice nurses should actively look for (and record) signs of personal growth in bereaved individuals, illustrated by statements such as 'I'm more tolerant of others than I used to be' and 'I don't let little things bother me like I used to'. In this context, Moyle Wright and Hogan also reflect on the DPM, and the importance of recognizing that even though there may be signs that the bereaved individual is coping, this does not mean that grief has ended.

Bruce (2007) discusses the impact of the pain of loss on health professionals. She identifies several key issues which arise from the nature of the relationship between the health and social care professional and their patient. 'A health and social care professional may say inwardly, "You've engaged me. I've invested myself in you. Now you're leaving"'. Then, there can be the narcissistic injury of, 'My job was to heal you, but I can't, and that feels terrible'. Frustrated altruistic strivings may include, 'I'm in this business to give life and to help others, so my energies must go to the living, not the dying'. There may be personal issues that are brought to the surface, or a crisis of faith brought on by particular circumstances: 'This one is too close to home!' or 'Why this, God?' It may be a matter of grief overload, as observed in health and social care professionals working in hospice or emergency trauma situations: 'Now this is just too much!' (Bruce, 2007: pp. 38-9). Any of these could, in the patient's eyes, lead staff to do exactly what they fear most – to withdraw emotionally and physically when the patient is most in need. These pressures exacerbate the potential for problematic grief experiences in health and social carers.

In order to cope with the grief when patients die, Bruce (2007) recommends that health and social care professionals need both time alone and time to share their feelings with others, as well as rest, relaxation, nourishment and diversion from the exhaustion of grief. These needs encompass the two arms of loss and restoration orientations. Many of the same bereavement facilities available to families can be of benefit to staff. Social support and counselling are important factors in enabling health and social care workers to cope with their job stressors. Counselling services for nurses are offered by the Royal College of Nursing and all NHS Trusts are required to provide counselling facilities for their staff.

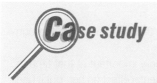

Case study

Pretending it's not going to happen…

Mr Taylor is a 67 year-old man who has been admitted to the oncology unit for symptom management. He was diagnosed with lung cancer a year ago, which was treated initially by radiotherapy. The treatment was only successful for a short time before he was diagnosed with extensive spread to other organs. He is now in the advanced stages of the disease and receiving palliative care. Mr Taylor had been admitted to hospital on this occasion by his GP for management of his pain and other symptoms but when assessed was found to be very near the end of life. Mr Taylor expressed a wish for the staff to be honest with him but also asked that they explain his condition and situation to his wife and family, adding that his wife had been completely in denial of his failing condition for some weeks. He had tried to get her to speak about their situation but she refused

saying he had to be more positive. He said this was not an unusual reaction from her but part of his concern was that their two children, who were now married with children, had moved to Australia. They had hoped to visit, with a view to joining them in a new life out there but this would now be impossible. He and his wife had been married 45 years and he told them she coped by not facing issues until they became a crisis and then she still needed a lot of support to get through them. He was anticipating her loss as well as his own loss of dreams by trying to put help in place for her before he died. By telling staff that he thought they were more experienced, of his dilemma, he thought they would be able to support her better following his death if they knew how she usually reacted to difficult situations.

1 What can the health and social care staff do to make the patient feel at ease?

2 What could the staff do to support the wife of the dying patient?

3 How can the bereaved carer be supported following the death?

Health Care Professional

Counsellor specializing in palliative care

A difficult situation

'When I arrived at the ward the charge nurse was annoyed as she had tasked one of her staff nurses with telling a lady her husband was dying. The conversation had not gone well and as a counsellor I had been asked in to support the family. My first thought was to gather the facts before meeting the patient or family as I had not previously been involved in counselling them. I asked the staff nurse who had been caring for the patient what had been said to his wife, and was aware the nurse was agitated. I explained that I wasn't there to organize the nursing staff in any way, merely to understand what had happened to the patient and their family, and so try to help them. The staff nurse began to cry saying how terrible she felt that she had made a mess of what she knew to be a difficult time for the family, and though she had tried to explain to senior colleagues that she had no experience in this sort of situation, she still felt that she had to go through with the situation.

Whilst my role was to help the patient, it also seemed really important at that time to support the staff nurse as not only had this situation a detrimental effect on her, but it had raised personal memories which she found distressing. I spent some time with her and arranged to meet her again later that week for a personal counselling session.'

KEY POINTS

● Health and social care staff can ease grief by communicating gently and clearly, listening and giving time for the bereaved person to take in the news about the patient, then giving practical advice.

● Whilst not disguising your own feelings, do not burden the bereaved with them, or attempt to justify the situation.

● When patients die, health and social care staff do need support too, needing time alone and with others to share their grief and process it. Counselling should be available.

CONCLUSIONS

Bereavement almost always leads to grief, although the extent of grieving is variable. Stage theories, suggest that feelings such as numbness and denial are followed by anger, despair and depression. Initially, bereaved individuals feel as though they cannot cope but, over time, most come to terms with their loss and reorganize their lives. The DPM suggests that a bereaved individual's responses oscillate between loss-orientation and restoration-orientation, with both being important in coping. Grief may result in a range of physical, behavioural, cognitive and emotional responses. For some individuals, the cultural demands of mourning, such as the funeral, are helpful although this differs for instance between men and women. Other differences in grieving arise as a result of the nature of the death (for example whether it was traumatic or was expected) and whether the individual has suffered many losses.

A grieving response can also occur in advance of death, for example in carers looking after patients with Alzheimer's disease. This anticipatory grieving can be very prolonged and distressing but does not necessarily prepare the grieving individual for the death when it does come.

Children's understanding of death develops slowly. Nevertheless, they are entitled to the opportunity to grieve.

Health and social care staff are regularly faced with trying to assist bereaved individuals. Being initially calm and accepting allows bereaved individuals the opportunity to express their immediate feelings if they wish.

Subsequently, being prepared to continue to listen and offering practical advice and reassurance are key roles. Eventually, formal services may be offered to bereaved individuals to help them to cope. The vigilance of health and social care staff to potential problems is important at this stage.

Finally, health and social care staff themselves may experience grief at the loss of patients and resources to assist in coping with the stresses of professional life are available.

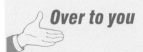

Over to you

Imagine a child who is in hospital awaiting treatment, whose parent is killed. They haven't said 'goodbye' and cannot attend the funeral. What emotions are they likely to experience and what assistance might they need? How would their grief differ if they were 4- or 7 years-old?

RAPID RECAP

Check your progress so far by working through each of the following questions.

1 How does the idea proposed by Worden (1991) differ from the stage processes described by Kübler-Ross and Parkes and why might Worden's approach be more useful?

2 What is the Dual Process Model and what advantages does it have over earlier explanations of grief?

3 a Identify four differences between the grieving of men and women.

   b Will all men and women differ in these ways?

   c In what ways is the experience of bereaved children similar to and different from that of adults?

4 The problem pages of magazines often describe the misery of people who care for a relative with a progressive disease, such as multiple sclerosis, who feel as though they are grieving before their relative has even died. How would you explain what they were experiencing if you were asked to do so by a hospital visitor expressing similar concerns?

If you have difficulty with any of the questions, read through the section again to refresh your understanding before moving on.

KEY REFERENCES

Other references are listed on the supporting website.

Almack, K., Seymour, J. and Bellamy, G. (2010) Exploring the Impact of Sexual Orientation on Experiences and the Impact of Sexual Orientation on Experiences and Concerns about End of Life care on Bereavement for Lesbian, Gay and Bisexual Older People, Sociology, 44

Dyregrov, K., Nordanger, D. and Dyregrov, A. (2003) Predictors of psychosocial stress after suicide, SIDS and accidents. *Death Studies*, 27: 143–165.

Lund, D.A., Utz, R., Caserta, M.S. and de Vries, B. (2008) Humor, Laughter & Happiness in the Daily Lives of Recently Bereaved Spouses. *Omega (Westport)*. 2008 ; 58(2): 87–105.

NHS The Route to Success in end of life care – achieving quality for lesbian, gay, bisexual and transgender people

NMC STANDARDS FOR PRE-REGISTRATION NURSING EDUCATION (2010)

Chapter title and learning outcomes

Chapter title and learning outcomes	Domain	Competency
General	Professional values	9. All nurses must appreciate the value of evidence in practice, be able to understand and appraise research, apply relevant theory and research findings to their work, and identify areas for further investigation.
2 Communication in the health care setting • Recognize the roles of communication in the health care setting. • Discuss factors affecting successful communication, evaluate interactions and suggest ways to improve communication. • Understand the importance of non-spoken aspects of communication. • Describe psychological factors that affect and enhance communication in a health care setting.	Communication and interpersonal skills	1. Build partnerships and therapeutic relationships. 2. Use a range of communication skills and technologies to support person-centred care and enhance quality and safety. 3. Use the full range of communication methods, including verbal, non-verbal and written, to acquire, interpret and record their knowledge and understanding of people's needs. 4. Recognize when people are anxious or in distress and respond effectively. 5. Use therapeutic principles to engage, maintain and, where appropriate, disengage from professional caring relationships, and must always respect professional boundaries. 8. Respect individual rights to confidentiality.
3 Psychology and the individual in health care settings • Outline how different personality types affect people in health care settings. • Understand what Emotional Intelligence is and how it affects people who work in health care settings. • Appreciate the difference between empathy and sympathy and outline how empathy affects people who work in health care settings. • Outline what Compassion Fatigue is and how it affects people who work in health care settings.	Communication and interpersonal skills Nursing practice and decision-making	5. Recognize when people are anxious or in distress and respond effectively. 4. Ascertain and respond to the physical, social and psychological needs of people.

4 Social interactions in the health care settings ● Outline causes of aggression in people and describe research into aggression in health care settings. ● Explain ways in which aggression can be dealt with in health care settings. ● Describe what prejudice is and how it could develop in people. ● Outline theories of prejudice. ● Appreciate how health care professionals' own prejudices might affect them in health care settings. ● Outline ways to tackle prejudice and apply them to health care settings.	Communication and interpersonal skills	5. Recognize when people are anxious or in distress and respond effectively, using therapeutic principles, to promote their well-being, manage personal safety and resolve conflict practise in a holistic, non-judgemental, caring and sensitive manner that avoids assumptions, supports social inclusion; recognizes and respects individual choice; and acknowledges diversity. Where necessary, they must challenge inequality, discrimination and exclusion from access to care.
	Nursing practice and decision-making	9. Be able to recognize when a person is at risk and in need of extra support and protection and take reasonable steps to protect them from abuse.
	Leadership, management and teamworking	4. Be self-aware and recognize how their own values, principles and assumptions may affect their practice.
5 Explaining and changing health care behaviour ● Define health behaviours and health habits. ● Discuss primary prevention. ● Describe and evaluate models of health behaviour. ● Discuss how models can be used to improve health behaviours. ● Develop and test a health intervention.	Communication and interpersonal skills	6. Take every opportunity to encourage health-promoting behaviour through education, role modelling and effective communication. 5. Understand public health principles, priorities and practice in order to recognize and respond to the major causes and social determinants of health, illness and health inequalities. They must use a range of information and data to assess the needs of people, groups, communities and populations, and work to improve health, well-being and experiences of health care; secure equal access to health screening, health promotion and health care; and promote social inclusion.
	Nursing practice and decision-making	7. Understand public health principles, priorities and practice in order to recognize and respond to the major causes and social determinants of health, illness and health inequalities. 8. Provide educational support, facilitation skills and therapeutic nursing interventions to optimize health and well-being. They must promote self-care and management whenever possible, helping people to make choices about their health care needs, involving families and carers where appropriate, to maximize their ability to care for themselves.

(Continued)

Chapter title and learning outcomes	Domain	Competency
6 Adherence to treatment ● Explain what is meant by patient non-adherence. ● Describe and evaluate methods for assessing adherence. ● Explain patient-related factors that help to understand why patients may not follow instructions given to them by health professionals. ● Explain practitioner-related factors that help to understand why patients may not follow instructions given to them by health professionals. ● Identify and justify good practice that would help patients to understand, remember and act on advice.	Nursing practice and decision-making	8. Provide educational support, facilitation skills and therapeutic nursing interventions to optimize health and well-being. They must promote self-care and management whenever possible, helping people to make choices about their health care needs, involving families and carers where appropriate, to maximize their ability to care for themselves. 10. Evaluate their care to improve clinical decision-making, quality and outcomes, using a range of methods, amending the plan of care, where necessary, and communicating changes to others.
7 Stress ● Define stress. ● Discuss biological and psychological explanations of stress. ● Describe research into the links between stress and health. ● Describe sources of stressors for patients and health care professionals. ● Identify biological, social and psychological factors that can increase an individual's experience of stress. ● Identify ways in which stress can affect social behaviour and performance. ● Describe and evaluate stress management strategies that could be used by patients and health care professionals.	Communication and interpersonal skills Nursing practice and decision-making	5. Recognize when people are anxious or in distress and respond effectively, using therapeutic principles, to promote their well-being, manage personal safety and resolve conflict practise in a holistic, non-judgemental, caring and sensitive manner that avoids assumptions, supports social inclusion; recognizes and respects individual choice; and acknowledges diversity. Where necessary, they must challenge inequality, discrimination and exclusion from access to care. 2. Possess a broad knowledge of the structure and functions of the human body, and other relevant knowledge from the life, behavioural and social sciences as applied to health, ill-health, disability, ageing and death. They must have an in-depth knowledge of common physical and mental health problems and treatments in their own field of practice, including co-morbidity and physiological and psychological vulnerability. Carry out comprehensive, systematic nursing assessments that take account of relevant physical, social, cultural, psychological, spiritual, genetic and environmental factors.

8 Pain		
• Describe pain in terms of its physiology and psychology. • Describe and evaluate the ways that pain can be measured. • Understand the factors affecting the perception of pain. • Describe and evaluate explanations of theories of pain. • Describe methods of pain relief and relate them to theories of pain.		7. Be able to recognize and interpret signs of normal and deteriorating mental and physical health and respond promptly to maintain or improve the health and comfort of the service user, acting to keep them and others safe. 8. Provide educational support, facilitation skills and therapeutic nursing interventions to optimize health and well-being. They must promote self-care and management whenever possible, helping people to make choices about their health care needs, involving families and carers where appropriate, to maximize their ability to care for themselves.
	Communication and interpersonal skills	5. Recognize when people are anxious or in distress and respond effectively, using therapeutic principles, to promote their well-being, manage personal safety and resolve conflict practise in a holistic, non-judgemental, caring and sensitive manner that avoids assumptions, supports social inclusion; recognizes and respects individual choice; and acknowledges diversity. Where necessary, they must challenge inequality, discrimination and exclusion from access to care.
	Nursing practice and decision-making	2. Possess a broad knowledge of the structure and functions of the human body, and other relevant knowledge from the life, behavioural and social sciences as applied to health, ill-health, disability, ageing and death. They must have an in-depth knowledge of common physical and mental health problems and treatments in their own field of practice, including co-morbidity and physiological and psychological vulnerability. 3. Carry out comprehensive, systematic nursing assessments that take account of relevant physical, social, cultural, psychological, spiritual, genetic and environmental factors, in partnership with service users and others through interaction, observation and measurement. 7. Be able to recognize and interpret signs of normal and deteriorating mental and physical health and respond promptly to maintain or improve the health and comfort of the service user, acting to keep them and others safe.

(Continued)

Chapter title and learning outcomes

	Domain	Competency
9 Bereavement and grief ● Describe common experiences of bereaved individuals and the tasks of the grieving process. ● Understand differences in the grieving process between individuals, including social and cultural differences. ● Explain the experience of grieving from different theoretical perspectives. ● Identify ways in which bereaved individuals and health care staff can be supported when a patient dies.	Professional values	3. Support and promote the health, well-being, rights and dignity of people, groups, communities and populations. These include people whose lives are affected by ill-health, disability, ageing, death and dying. 4. Must work in partnership with service users, carers, groups, communities and organizations. They must manage risk, and promote health and well-being while aiming to empower choices that promote self-care and safety.
	Nursing practice and decision-making	1. Must use up-to-date knowledge and evidence to assess, plan, deliver and evaluate care, communicate findings, influence change and promote health and best practice. They must make person-centred, evidence-based judgements and decisions, in partnership with others involved in the care process, to ensure high quality care. They must be able to recognize when the complexity of clinical decisions requires specialist knowledge and expertise, and consult or refer accordingly. 4. Ascertain and respond to the physical, social and psychological needs of people, groups and communities. They must then plan, deliver and evaluate safe, competent, person-centred care in partnership with them, paying special attention to changing health needs during different life stages, including progressive illness and death, loss and bereavement.

APPENDIX

ANSWERS TO RAPID RECAP QUESTIONS

CHAPTER 1

1 What is the difference between a behavourist explanation and a cognitive one?

A behaviourist explanation uses learning, e.g. operant or classical conditioning or social learning to explain a phenomenon, whereas a cognitive explanation focuses on the individual's information processing, such as their memory or the language they use.

2 What did Freud suggest could control our behaviour that made his explanations different from other theories?

The unconscious.

3 Why do psychologists use statistics in their research?

They use descriptive statistics to illustrate averages or to indicate the spread of data and internal statistics so that they can be more sure about the likelihood that the results they have found could have arisen by chance.

CHAPTER 2

1 What is the communication cycle?

The process by which we communicate. A message is transmitted from one person (the sender) to another (the recipient) and the cycle is completed by feedback from the recipient back to the sender.

2 What is meant by 'patient-centred' and 'doctor-centred' approaches to interaction?

Patient-centred means treating the patient as an individual, rather than a commodity. The patient is an active participant in the interaction and can influence the outcome. Doctor-centred means the practitioner asking the patient questions about their condition, which allows the provision of a diagnosis and appropriate treatment. Communication is two-way but is directed by one of the participants.

3 What does the acronym SURETY stand for?

Sit at an angle to the client
Uncross your legs
Relax
Eye contact
Touch
Your intuition

CHAPTER 3

1 Outline how someone's personality might affect their work in a health and social care setting.

It can affect people in many different ways. EI is about perceiving, realizing, understanding and managing emotions in a health and social care setting. This can be used to help patients come to terms with their health issues and allow health and social care professionals to understand how a patient may be feeling. These two ideas can help a patient break through the psychological barrier with regards to any health issues they have. Empathy can also be beneficial as it is about the ability to share someone else's feelings by imagining what it would be like to be in their situation – this will also help to strengthen any professional-patient bond.

2 What is Emotional Intelligence?

A person's ability to monitor their own emotions and the emotions of others correctly.

3 What is the difference between empathy and sympathy? How can empathy affect workers in health and social care settings?

Empathy is the ability to share someone else's feelings by imagining what it would be like to be in their situation. This may be because you have experienced something similar yourself. Therefore, it is more about *relating* with a patient in a health and social care setting. Remember that **sympathy** is just about acknowledging someone else's emotional issues and providing comfort based on that. Empathy allows health and social care professionals to understand what the patient is going through but it may decline over time and make some people emotionally 'burnout'.

4 **Can Compassion Fatigue affect workers in health and social care settings? Justify your answer using evidence.**

Health and social care professionals experience both emotional and physical fatigue/tiredness due to an over usage of empathy when dealing with patients' problems and conditions. The over use of empathy 'builds up over time' so it is cumulative and can ultimately lead to professional **burnout** when the person simply 'cannot face the emotional aspects linked to work'. Studies have shown (e.g. Craig and Sprang, 2010) that exposure to stressful situations involving patients that require some level of compassion, leads to increased burnout as the health and social care professional has to continually deal with this (even on a daily basis).

CHAPTER 4

1 **Identify two causes of aggression.**

Testosterone and Social Learning Theory.

2 **What are the four stages of Social Learning Theory?**

Attention, Retention, Reproduction and Motivation.

3 **How can prejudice affect workers in a health and social care setting?**

It can affect them in many ways. Nurses may feel prejudiced towards a patient who needs treatment for something that they do not agree with (e.g. recreational drug user). This may affect how they interact with the patient. This has been seen in head trauma patients and also obese patients. Also, nurses may have implicit prejudice, which means they are unconsciously prejudiced against a certain type of patient and may not realize that they are treating them in a negative way.

4 **Outline one way in which we can reduce prejudice.**

Have contact with the stereotyped group via Expectation: The person who knows that there is about to be some interaction between themselves and a stereotyped out-group member. Adjustment: If the meeting is on 'equal terms' then the whole process should be a positive one. Generalization: The positive experience was probably not expected (after all we are talking about prejudice!) but it should leave an impression that other members of the stereotyped group are the same and prejudice begins to be reduced.

CHAPTER 5

1   **What influences behaviour change according to the health belief model**

    The HBM identifies five core beliefs. These are:

    Perceived vulnerability – the individual's assessment of the risk that they will be affected by the condition.

    Perceived seriousness – the individual's assessment of how bad the effect will be if they are affected.

    Perceived barriers – aspects of the situation that disincline the individual to take action.

    Perceived benefits – possible gains for the individual.

    Cues to action – an immediate trigger for acting healthily.

2   **What are the key elements in the theory of planned behaviour.**

    The theory of planned behaviour proposes that actions, such as health behaviours, are determined by a combination of behavioural intention (deciding to achieve a goal) and perceived behavioural control (believing that you can or cannot perform a behaviour).

3   **How does an individual progress through the stages of change according to the transtheoretical model and what role do the processes of change play in their progress?**

    Through precontemplation, contemplation, preparation, action and maintenance followed by either termination or relapse (the latter leading to a return to precontemplation). The processes of change are the covert and overt activities that an individual uses to progress through the stages.

4   **The following factors could affect an individual who is thinking about giving up smoking: the existence of many non-smoking restaurants; the belief that smoky clothes are unpleasant; a desire to combat the effects of smoking on their asthma; the knowledge that they can stop themselves from starting again once they have said they've given up. Explain which of these factors would relate to each of these models**

    Health Belief model:
    Benefits – easier to access non-smoking environments than smoking ones, not smelling, reduced asthma symptoms.

    Theory of planned behaviour:
    Behavioural intention – the existence of many non-smoking restaurants; the belief that smoky clothes are unpleasant; desire to combat the effects of smoking on their asthma.

    Perceived behavioural control – the knowledge that they can stop themselves from starting again once they have said they've given up.

Transtheoretical model:
Contemplation – consider benefits of not smelling and reducing asthma symptoms, Preparation – finding out about non-smoking restaurants, believing that avoiding relapse is possible.

CHAPTER 6

1 **What are the differences between the Behavioural and Cognitive models of compliance?**

The Behavioural model targets the actual behaviour side of non-adherence whereas the Cognitive model targets the thought processes behind why we do not adhere to treatment.

2 **Explain how personality might affect adherence to treatment.**

There are many different ways in which personality can affect adherence. People who have traits like Agreeableness and Conscientiousness tend to adhere more than those who are Neurotic.

3 **Outline two ways in which we could improve adherence to treatment.**

The first one is Text Messaging: this can be used to send encouraging messages to people once they have stuck to a health programme and it can also be used to motivate them if they begin to find adherence difficult. The second one is: Memory Intervention. A very recent strategy includes the following: Emphasize routine, Develop cues, Elaborate the action, Do it now, Implement intentions and Teach – ask – wait – ask again – wait – ask again.

CHAPTER 7

1 **Outline a biological mechanism involved in stress.**

One mechanism is the hypothalamic–pituitary–adrenocortical axis. If the stressor is not removed the body responds differently via cortisol breaking down fatty tissue, releasing soluble fats and stimulating the release of glucose from the liver so that the muscles can obtain more energy from the blood. In addition, Aldosterone increases blood pressure, maintaining the body ready for action. Finally, Thyroxine increases the body's metabolic rate. This means that the stressed person can extract energy from food more quickly.

2 **Outline the transactional model of stress (Lazarus).**

Lazarus and Folkman (1984) suggest that this process of determining whether a situation is threatening, challenging or harmful is one of appraisal. Our initial impression or primary appraisal of the situation generates emotions based on a threat, or the anticipation of harm, like fear, anxiety or worry. Then when harm, or damage has already happened we may feel disgust, disappointment, anger or sadness. As we challenge the stressor, we generate an appraisal of anticipation or excitement. Following the initial appraisal, a secondary appraisal is made. This is the formation of an impression about one's ability to cope with the situation.

3 **How can stressors affect you in the workplace?**

It can affect people in many ways like by affecting health (like increased blood pressure), social behaviours (like getting angry more easily) and overall job satisfaction.

4 **Describe and evaluate one way we could cope with stress.**

Mindfulness-Based Stress Reduction. It incorporates meditation, yoga and mind-body exercises to teach people how to cope with stress caused by lifestyle and work. There appears to be some evidence to suggest it works: Nyklíček *et al.* (2013) and Wolever *et al.*

CHAPTER 8

1 **Describe one way in which pain is measured in a clinical setting and one way in which it can be measured for the purposes of research.**

Clinical setting: Self-reporting, where the patient records their pain in words as a description or on a diagram, indicating the location and intensity.

Research: Cold-pressor test, where the participant has to keep their hand submerged in ice cold water for as long as they can, the time elapsed before the hand is removed indicating their pain tolerance.

2 **Too much work on a computer or reading a book can lead to an eye-strain headache. How would the gate control theory of pain account for the effectiveness of rubbing one's eyes to relieve the pain?**

The physical effect of rubbing the eyes stimulates the large (A-beta) nerve fibres that send signals up to the gate in the spinal cord and close it. This prevents perception of the pain of the headache.

3 **Vinar (1969) reported a case study of an individual who had become dependent upon a placebo. Use the idea of expectation to explain how this situation might have arisen.**

The belief that a treatment will relieve pain results in pain reduction. If the patient had been taking the placebo for a long time and had not experienced pain (because it was no longer necessary), they could have built up an expectation that they would suffer if they stopped taking it. The patient's absence of pain while taking the placebo would have confirmed their belief that they needed it to be pain-free.

CHAPTER 9

1 **How does the idea proposed by Worden (1991) differ from the stage processes described by Kübler-Ross and Parkes and why might Worden's approach be more useful?**

By stating that it is more useful to identify the tasks to be achieved through mourning:

- accepting the reality of the loss
- working through the pain
- adjusting to the absence of the deceased from the environment
- moving forward in life.

Worden's approach might be more useful because it allows for individual differences that will arise in the exact stages or feelings that each person experiences and the order in which they happen.

2 **What is the Dual Process Model and what advantages does it have over earlier explanations of grief?**

The dual process model proposes that in grief we alternate between an orientation of loss in which we focus on the loved one we miss and one of restoration in which we focus on coping with the new situation. This theory enable us to explain why people's experience of grief can fluctuate over the short term and offers ways to help people to gain relief from the stress of the loss orientation by accepting the need for restoration and, conversely, accepting the need for the sadness of grief.

3 **a. Identify four differences between the grieving of men and women.**

Four from:

- Women tend to display more overt grief than men.
- Women are more likely to suffer obsessional grief.
- Women are more likely to benefit from attending a funeral.
- Women are less likely to turn to alcohol than men.
- Women describe feelings of abandonment whereas men describe feeling dismembered.
- Women tend to feel angry and cry whereas men feel 'choked up' and guilty.
- Men make a faster social recovery than women but take longer to overcome the emotional consequences.

b. Will all men and women differ in these ways?

No, there will be individual, cultural and societal differences as well as gender-related ones.

c. In what ways is the experience of bereaved children similar to and different from that of adults?

Bereaved children suffer many of the same emotions, of guilt, anger, numbness and depression as adults. However they differ from adults in their less predictable response and their differing understanding of the concept of death, depending on their age.

4 **The problem pages of magazines often describe the misery of people who care for a relative with a progressive disease, such as multiple sclerosis, who feel as though they are grieving before their relative has even died. How would you explain what they were experiencing if you were asked to do so by a hospital visitor expressing similar concerns?**

I would explain that they are experiencing anticipatory grieving. They identify feelings of loss that resemble bereavement while the individual is still alive because the person they once knew no longer exists. They may experience anger, fear of abandonment as the relationship deteriorates, depression and sleeplessness. Anticipatory grief can also lead to an increased risk of catching infections but if carers themselves have good social support, they tend to cope better. In addition, emotions including sadness, feeling overwhelmed or trapped, frustration and guilt may be felt. These will be distressing but are common in this situation.

INDEX

CREDITS

All Figures and artwork other than those listed below, are the authors' own work.

Figure 1.1 p. 12 – Fully adapted from Aubert et al 1998

Figure 1.3 p. 13 – Data sourced from OECD

Figure 1.4 p. 13 – Fully adapted from Beaumont (2013)

Figure 1.5 p. 14 – Data sourced from Health survey for England. Health and Social Care
Centre (2011)

Figure 4.1 p. 80 – Fully adapted from Farrell et al 2010

Figure 7.2 p. 171 – Fully adapted from Elmar Gräßel and Raffaela Adabbo (2011) 'Perceived Burden of Informal Caregivers of a Chronically Ill Older Family Member Burden in the Context of the Transactional Stress Model of Lazarus and Folkman' *GeroPsych*, 24 (3), 2011, 143–154

Figure 8.2 p. 198 – McGill Pain Questionnaire – Fully adapted from Melzack (1983)

Figure 8.6 p. 209 – Fully adapted from Godfrey, 2005

Figure 8.7 p. 211 – Fully adapted from Godfrey, 2005

Figure 8.8 p. 220 – Fully adapted from Melzack (2001)

All images are © Shutterstock

Paul Mason

UNDERSTANDING COMPUTER SAFETY

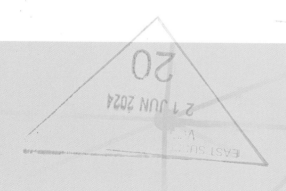

Raintree is an imprint of Capstone Global Library Limited, a company incorporated in England and
Wales having its registered office at 7 Pilgrim Street, London, EC4V 6LB – Registered company number:
6695582

www.raintreepublishers.co.uk
myorders@raintreepublishers.co.uk

Edited by Linda Staniford and Chris Harbo
Designed by Richard Parker and Tim Bond
Original illustrations © Capstone Global Library 2015
Illustrated by Nigel Dobbyn (Beehive Illustration)
Picture research by Jo Miller
Production by Victoria Fitzgerald
Originated by Capstone Global Library Ltd
Printed and bound in China by CTPS

ISBN 978 1 406 28977 0 (hardback)
18 17 16 15 14
10 9 8 7 6 5 4 3 2 1

ISBN 978 1 406 28982 4 (paperback)
19 18 17 16
10 9 8 7 6 5 4 3 2 1

British Library Cataloguing in Publication Data
A full catalogue record for this book is available from the British Library.

Acknowledgements
We would like to thank the following for permission to reproduce photographs:

Alamy: ©imageBROKER, 16, ©Isabelle Plasschaert, 39, ©Marmaduke St. John, 40, © maximimages.
com, 17 left and right, ©NUAGE, 31, ©Oote Boe Photography, 20; Corbis: ©Ann Summa, 4, Blend
Images/©Kevin Dodge, 18, ©Stefanie Grewel, 42; Dreamstime©Dragonimages, 15; Getty Images:
Altrendo/altrendo images, 5, flickr Editorial/Moment Mobile /Hattanas Kumcha, 24; iStockphoto:
©daizuoxin, 14, ©PacoRomero, 7, © Veesaandijc, 6, ©Yuri_Arcurs, 8; Shutterstock:areya_ann, 37, Alexey
Boldin, 13, Blend Images, 26, Goodluz, 36, Martin Novak, 22, Monkey Business Images, 43, racorn, 25,
tab62, 30, T.W. van Urk, 10, Viktoria Kazakova, cover; SuperStock: agefotostock, 38.
Design Elements: Shutterstock: HuntThomas, vectorlib.com (throughout)

We would like to thank Andrew Connell for his invaluable help in the preparation of this book.

Every effort has been made to contact copyright holders of material reproduced in this book. Any
omissions will be rectified in subsequent printings if notice is given to the publisher.

All the internet addresses (URLs) given in this book were valid at the time of going to press. However,
due to the dynamic nature of the internet, some addresses may have changed, or sites may have
changed or ceased to exist since publication. While the author and publisher regret any inconvenience
this may cause readers, no responsibility for any such changes can be accepted by either the author or
the publisher.